David Powers
McRae 302

human embryology

human embryology
a regional approach

M.J.T. FitzGerald, M.D., Ph.D., D. Sc.,
Professor and Chairman, Department of Anatomy, University College,
Galway, Ireland; Formerly Associate Professor, Department of
Biological Structure, University of Washington School of Medicine,
Seattle, Washington; Formerly Associate Professor, Department of
Anatomy, St. Louis University School of Medicine, St. Louis, Missouri;
Formerly Reader in Anatomy, University College, Cork, Ireland;
and Formerly Lecturer in Anatomy, St. Thomas's Hospital Medical
School, London, England

Medical Department
Harper & Row, Publishers
Hagerstown, Maryland
New York, San Francisco, London

78 79 80 81 82 83   10 9 8 7 6 5 4 3 2 1

Library of Congress Cataloging in Publication Data

Fitzgerald, M   J   T
    Human embryology.

    Includes bibliographies and index.
    1. Embryology, Human. I. Title. [DNLM:
1. Embryology. QS604 F554h]
QM601.F65   612.6′4   77–26077
ISBN 0–06–140824–7

He, too, has been changed
in his turn,
Transformed utterly:
A terrible beauty is born

Yeats

contents

preface

Any teacher who contemplates writing an Embryology textbook, of primary
interest to medical students, must first resolve some conflicts of interest. On the
one hand, the highly complex sequence of events that transforms the single
fertilized cell into a fully formed infant is manifestly important as a basis for an
understanding of adult anatomy. Secondly, the incidence of birth defects—of the
order of 5% of all live births—renders an appreciation of *abnormal*
developmental events relevant to later clinical training in obstetrics and
pediatrics. (The variety of malformations encountered in clinical practice is very
large: those of the heart and great vessels alone exceed one hundred.) On both
of these grounds a comprehensive treatment of the subject would seem to be
necessary.

On the other hand, the preclinical student has a great deal more than
Embryology to contend with. In Anatomy alone, he or she is also required to
master the relevant features of Topographic Anatomy, Histology, and Neurology.
When one adds to these Biochemistry, Physiology, Behavioral Science and
perhaps early patient contact, it becomes imperative to place Embryology in its
proper place in the total educational context. It is but a short step to the
conclusion that a textbook which introduces students to Embryology must
therefore contain enough—but just enough—information to provide for their
needs. The presentation must also be sufficiently clear to encourage a substantial
amount of the material to be understood by private reading. This book has
been written with these two considerations particularly in mind.

My aim has been to provide a straightforward account of human development,
to serve as a primary source of information to students approaching the subject
for the first time. The emphasis throughout is on normal development.
Malformations are also treated, but with the brevity which befits an introductory
work, and the short bibliographies refer to the interested reader to some recent
reviews and to older, classical accounts. Because the precise meaning of
embryologic terminology is crucial to learning, a glossary is included; it should
be referred to frequently as reading proceeds.

In any course in human anatomy it is desirable that the development of each
region of the body be considered in company with the program in topographical
(gross) anatomy. Accordingly, the format of this book departs from tradition
in presenting the salient features of Embryology on a *regional* basis. Separate
chapters describe the development of: spinal cord and body wall, the thoracic
organs, the abdominal and pelvic organs, and the head and neck. The text is

designed so that, following mastery of the early features of development in Chapters 1 to 8, one can read the subsequent chapters in any order of choice. A second advantage of the regional approach is that the description of the systems is completed within each region; this permits an immediate appreciation of the way in which the different systems impinge on one another as they develop.

The book will also be of interest to students of dentistry, and to Science students whose courses include instruction in human anatomy.

acknowledgments

First, I thank my wife, Maeve. Her suggestions and criticisms during the preparation of this book have been of enormous help.

The line drawings (except those I have signed) were rendered by Mrs. Hilary Gilmore. I am most grateful for her skill and understanding.

I thank my secretary, Miss Mary R. O'Donnell, for preparing several revisions of the text.

Most medical students do not have the opportunity to study sectioned embryos under the microscope. For this reason the line drawings have been supplemented by photographs of well-prepared sections. For permission to reproduce material from the Carnegie Institution of Embryology in Washington, D.C., I am indebted to Dr. J.D. Ebert; Dr. B. Boving assisted my study of the collection and Mr. Richard Grill made the photographic negatives. I am grateful to Dr. T.H. Shepard of the University of Washington School of Medicine, Seattle, for permission to study the collection of embryos in the Department of Pediatrics; Mr. George Reis of the Department of Biological Structure gave photographic assistance. At Cambridge University, Professor R.J. Harrison kindly allowed me to study the embryo collection in the Anatomy School, and Mr. J. Cash assisted in the provision of photographic negatives. Here, at Galway, Mr. Pierce Lalor did the final printing.

I am happy to acknowledge the encouragement and advice freely given by the Editorial, Art, and Production departments of Harper & Row, Publishers.

human embryology

Chapter 1

introduction

Human embryology is the science that is concerned with the prenatal development of man. The prenatal period commences at the moment of fertilization, when male and female sex cells unite to form the *zygote*—a unicellular organism that will give rise to a new individual. The event of birth is an arbitrary termination of this period; development continues, although at a progressively slower rate, until maturity. The complete developmental story of man is his *ontogeny*.

OVUM, EMBRYO, FETUS

Prenatal development continues for 40 weeks (about 280 days) from fertilization. It may be divided into three periods. The *period of the ovum* (two weeks) extends from fertilization to the completion of implantation in the wall of the uterus. The *embryonic period* extends from the beginning of the third week to the end of the eighth week of development. During this time the organ systems of the body are laid down and the placenta is constructed. The *fetal period* lasts from the beginning of the ninth week of gestation until full term; this is primarily a period of increase in size.

The appearance of malformations in a newborn child is usually due to interference with development in the embryonic or early fetal period, because interference before implantation will lead to death of the ovum, and during the late fetal period it will tend to cause only stunting of growth.

The term *conceptus* is taken to mean the product of conception. It denotes both the embryoblast and the trophoblast, and their derivatives.

PATTERN OF EARLY DEVELOPMENT

Some advance knowledge of the pattern of early development will be found helpful for the purpose of orientation. The principal events are shown in Figure 1-1; they are as follows:

After fertilization the zygote (**A**) travels along the oviduct to the uterus. As it travels it divides repeatedly to form a ball of cells (**B**) called the *morula* (*morula* means a mulberry). The morula resolves into two cell groups (**C**). One group secures nourishment for the embryo by burrowing into the wall of the uterus to tap the maternal blood vessels there. It is

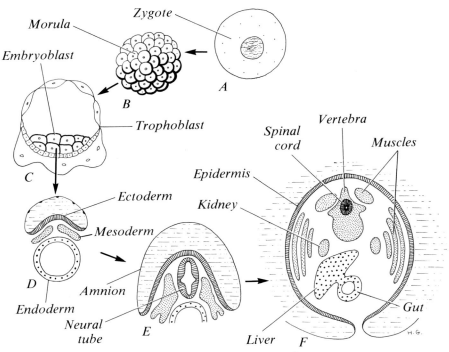

FIG. 1-1. Summary of early development.

known as the *trophoblast* (*trophe,* nutrition; *blast,* generative); the complex organ of nourishment that it erects is the *placenta.* The second cell group is the *embryoblast;* it produces all the tissues of the embryo. The embryoblast gives rise to three cell layers—the *ectoderm,* the *mesoderm,* and the *endoderm* (**D**). The ectoderm invests the embryo and forms the epidermis of the skin; it gives rise also to the *neural tube,* from which the nervous system is derived. Its margins give attachment to the *amnion,* a fluid-filled sac that develops to surround and protect the embryo (**E**). The mesoderm is laid down on each side of the midline. It produces the various connective tissues of the body, and it forms much of the urogenital system. The endoderm forms the epithelial lining of the alimentary tract. The lungs, liver, pancreas, and other organs develop from the gut epithelium at appropriate levels (**F**).

INDUCTION

The manner in which the first elements—the *primordia,* or *buds*—of the various organs are derived from the parent germ layers is of particular interest to the embryologist. What, for example, causes the ectoderm to give rise to the neural tube, the mesoderm to the kidneys, or the endoderm to the liver? The evidence from experimental embryology indicates that cell groups of different germ layers (or, within a germ layer, of different properties) interact with one another to influence their course of development. This is the phenomenon of *induction,* and it depends upon the *organizer* influence of one cell group acting upon the reactive potential, or *competence,* of another. Thus it appears that the mesoderm (together with the notochord) exerts an organizing influence upon the overlying ectoderm, which responds by forming the neural tube. The neural tube in turn organizes the developing vertebrae to contribute protective neural arches to surround it. The mechanism of induction is uncertain; it may depend on physical interaction between cell groups, on chemical diffusion, or on alteration of the intercellular matrix.

GROWTH AND DIFFERENTIATION

Embryonic development comprises the twin processes of growth and differentiation. *Growth* is the increase in embryonic size produced by the multiplication, secretion, and enlargement of cells. *Differentiation* (literally, the development of differences) is the progressive increase in structural complexity brought about by the acquisition of special characters by various cell groups. Differentiation of a cell group—for example, cells destined to form muscle or cartilage—is molecular at first; that is to say, the cells do not assume at once the visible characteristic of the tissue that they will form. This preliminary phase of *chemodifferentiation* leads to the manufacture of products characteristic of the cell type— myofibrils or cartilaginous ground substance, in our examples. The visible appearance and progression of cellular differentiation is known as *histogenesis, i.e.,* the development of tissue. Later still, tissues of more than one kind come together to form the body organs; this is the process of *organogenesis.*

The growth curve of all multicellular organisms, be they plant or animal, is sigmoid in shape; following a relatively slow initial increase, growth accelerates rapidly for a time, then slows down as the organism approaches maturity. A representative curve of human growth, including the first postnatal year, is shown in Figure 1-2. Birth takes place at the steepest part of the total curve. However, there is some reduction in the fetal growth rate, associated with a reduced blood flow through the placenta, after the 36th week of gestation. Closer scrutiny of the neonatal period would reveal a transient loss of weight as the infant adapts to a terrestrial (as distinct from aquatic!) environment. This loss is usually recovered by the tenth postnatal day.

FIG. 1-2. Weight–age relationships in early development. (Adapted from Thompson, DW: On Growth and Form, Cambridge University Press, 1942)

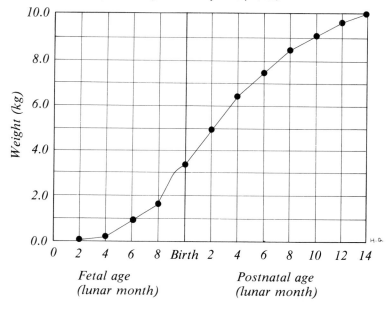

The growth curve of the whole organism is made up of the individual curves of its organs. Although the growth of the organs is again sigmoid, considerable differences are observed in their individual rates and time spans.

Figure 1-3 shows how the external appearance changes during the 30th–60th days after fertilization. The *somite period* of development is from the 20th–30th day. It is so called because, during this time, the mesoderm beside the neural tube breaks up into about 40 blocks called *somites,* which will form the vertebrae and the muscles of the trunk. The *branchial arches* and the *eye* appear during the somite period. The branchial arches are thickenings of the mesoderm in the sides and floor of the pharynx; they are homologous with the gill arches of fishes. The *limb buds* are visible at 30 days as tiny, blunt projections on the trunk. The *heart* is enormous; this is because it must pump blood through the extracorporeal circulation of the placenta as well as through the embryo itself.

At 40–50 days the large head reflects the rapid development of the brain. The limb buds have advanced and paddle-shaped expansions denote the future hands and feet. At 60 days differentiation is well advanced and the fetus is recognizably human.

The length of an embryo or fetus is a more reliable guide to its age than is its weight. The standard index is the *sitting height,* the distance from the crown of the head to the flexure of the rump. This measurement is known as the *crown–rump length* (Fig. 1-3). Average crown–rump values are given in Table 1-1.

TABLE 1-1. CROWN–RUMP LENGTH RELATED TO AGE

AGE (WEEKS)	LENGTH (MM)
4	5
5	8
6	12
8	23
12	56
16	110
20	160
24	200
28	240
32	280
36	310
40	350

FIG. 1-3. Changes in external form. (NOTE: The third and fourth figures are drawn to a reduced scale; actual size increases progressively.) Vertical line in third figure shows crown–rump length.

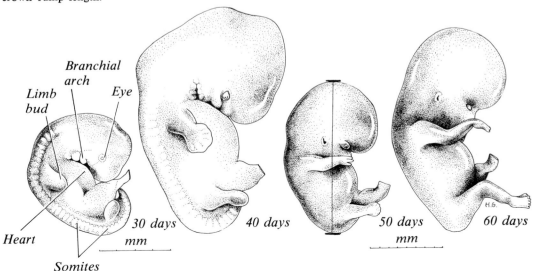

MITOSIS AND MEIOSIS

With a single exception, all animal cells multiply in the same manner, by *mitosis*. During mitosis the cytoplasm is halved, and each of the 46 nuclear chromosomes splits to provide a full and identical complement for each daughter cell. The single exception is the sex cell, or *germ cell* (*gamete*). Since the male and female germ cells contribute an equal number of chromosomes to the zygote, which has 46 chromosomes, a preliminary halving of the chromosome number is required. This is achieved by *meiosis*.

The two types of cell division are compared in Figure 1-4. For clarity, only four chromosomes are shown in each parent cell. The first column of the figure shows the events of mitosis. During interphase (the period between successive cell divisions) the cell doubles in size. The chromosomes are too attenuated to be seen with the light microscope, but they are known to become duplicated, the originals and their replicas being united along their whole length. During prophase the chromosomes split longitudinally into pairs of *chromatids* which are connected at one point (the *centromere*). In metaphase the chromatids move to the equatorial region. In telophase the chromatids separate to become the chromosomes of the two new cells.

Meiosis entails two cell divisions that together form a single sequence (central and right portions of Fig. 1-4). The interphase preceding the first division is similar to that of a somatic cell. During the prophase of the first division the chromosomes split (except at the centromeres) and homologous pairs of duplicated chromosomes approach and overlap one another. This affords opportunity for a variable amount of interchange of chromosomal segments (*crossover*). The first division concludes by the separation of the partly shuffled

FIG. 1-4. Mitosis and meiosis compared. **I**, interphase; **P**, prophase; **M**, metaphase; **T**, telophase.

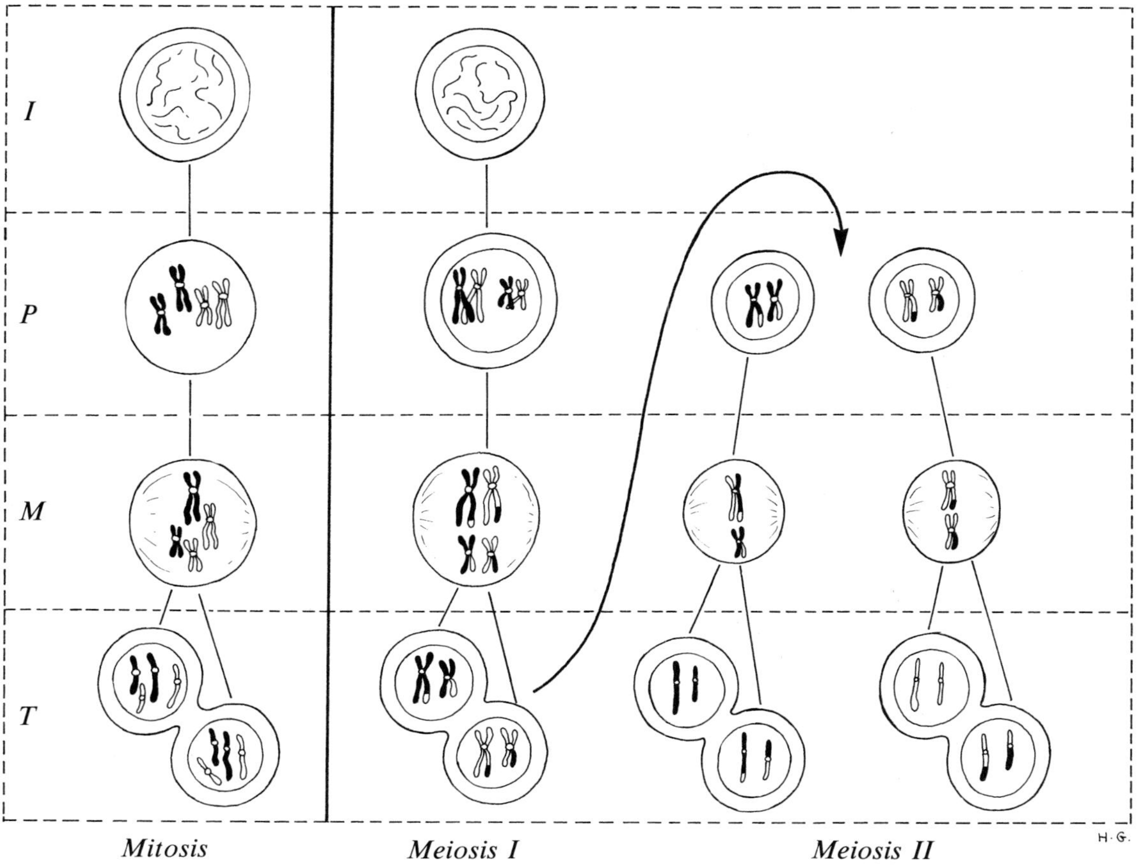

Mitosis   *Meiosis I*   *Meiosis II*

H·G·

homologues. The double-stranded chromosomes, *i.e.,* chromatid pairs, *still attached at the centromeres* pass to one or other daughter cell. The second division of meiosis merely completes the separation of the chromatid pairs. There is no significant interphase here because the chromosomes are already both duplicated and split. The chromatids separate at the centromeres and constitute the chromosomes of the offspring. The reduction of the chromosome number in meiosis has therefore been achieved by a double cell division; whereas the somatic cell has produced two cells, each containing 46 chromosomes, the sex cell has produced four gametes, each with 23 chromosomes.

CELL DEATH

The death of cell groups is a well-recognized feature of embryonic development. *Phylogenetic death* is observed in structures that are permanent in lower forms but are only vestigial in man. Such are the tubules of the pronephros, which is the permanent kidney of larval amphibia and of some bony fishes. Pronephric tubules can be detected in the cervical region of the human embryo for a few days, but they quickly die away. *Histogenetic death* occurs during tissue reorganization. The death of cartilage during the process of ossification of a long bone and the later erosion of newly formed bone are examples. *Morphogenetic death* takes place during the reshaping of body parts. Its operation is well shown in the developing hands and feet; these are at first paddle-shaped, the primordia of the digits being joined by webs. The digits become defined by degeneration and resorption of the webs.

CONGENITAL MALFORMATIONS

A congenital malformation is a *gross structural deformity present at birth*. Its incidence is about 2.5% in all infants born. However, only half of these deformities are apparent at the time of delivery, most of the remainder coming to light during the first postnatal year. It is usual to use the terms "malformation," "abnormality," and "defect" interchangeably, and to reserve "anomaly" for a minor congenital disorder such as a deformed finger or earlobe. Anomalies are found in a further 2.5% of live-born infants.

Approximately one pregnancy in five ends in the spontaneous abortion of the newly implanted ovum. The figures cited in the preceding paragraph do not take into account the high incidence (about one-third) of malformations in these newly implanted ova.

Abnormal development is called *teratogenesis* (*teras,* monster), and *teratology* is the science that is concerned with its investigation.

A study carried out in Birmingham, England, gives the relative frequency of the more common malformations (McKeown and Record):

Club foot	19%
Cardiac abnormalities	18%
Spina bifida cystica	13%
Hydrocephalus	11%
Anencephaly	9%
Cleft lip/cleft palate	8%
Down's syndrome (mongolism)	7%

In the United States, congenital abnormalities account for 7% of deaths occurring in infants during their first year of life. Congenital heart diseases cause half and central nervous disorders 17% of these deaths.

ETIOLOGY

The assessment of the relative roles of heredity and environment in the causation of abnormalities presents many difficulties. Only some 20% of abnormalities can be assigned either to a genetic fault on the one hand, or to the effect of disease, drugs, and the like on the other. In the remaining 80% the genetic make-up of the embryo *predisposes* towards a particular abnormality the manifestation of which is precipitated by some environmental disturbance.

Teratogenic agents may act in many ways: 1) by altering the rate of cell proliferation, 2) by preventing normal synthesis of enzymes, 3) by altering cell surfaces so that cellular aggregation fails or is otherwise abnormal, 4) by altering the matrix so as to interfere with the normal movement of cells, or 5) by damaging the organizer capacity of cells, or the competence of cells to respond to organizers. Even in closely observed animal models it is often impossible to determine the locus of action of a particular teratogen.

Genetic Factors

Abnormal genes may be inherited from one or both parents, and they may be dominant or recessive. In the majority of the afflicted, however, a mendelian pattern of inheritance cannot be discerned; the abnormalities merely occur more frequently among relatives than in the general population. In those occurring among relatives, there may be a complex interplay between several genes. In this group of subjects occur the malformations listed in the Birmingham study.

Deformities due to abnormal dominant genes are rare. In most of these the skeleton is affected and the deformities include achondroplasia, arachnodactyly, craniocleidal dysostosis, and osteogenesis imperfecta. Any one of such conditions will appear in 50% of the offspring of the affected parent.

Abnormal recessive genes do not find expression unless inherited from both parents; in such instances the abnormality may be found in 25% of the offspring. Cystic fibrosis of the pancreas and Sprengel's deformity of the shoulder are examples.

Malformations involving abnormal distribution of entire chromosomes are considered in Chapter 2.

Genetic factors, when they are operative, are the *remote* cause (initiating agent) of malformations. Each gene locus is concerned with the synthesis of an enzyme or polypeptide; and the *immediate* cause, which results from the genetic abnormality, is a biochemical disturbance at cell or tissue level. Some such disturbances can be imitated by environmental factors operating directly on cell or tissue. Morphologically similar defects may therefore have the same immediate cause (a specific biochemical disturbance) but a quite different remote cause.

The Environment

Infections. The most dangerous known teratogenic organism is the virus of *German measles* (*rubella*). Contraction of the disease by the mother during the first month of pregnancy appears to carry about a 50% risk of producing a congenital abnormality; during the second month the risk is about 25% and during the third month about 7%. The virus tends to affect the developing eyes, heart, ears, and palate. The triad of congenital cataract, heart disease, and deafness have become known as the *rubella syndrome*.

Cytomegalovirus (CMV) infection is found all over the world. Like the rubella virus it passes through the placenta to infect the fetus. The CMV is found in 0.5–1% of newborn babies, and about 10% of these show signs of disease. It may cause deafness, mental retardation, epilepsy, liver disease, or cerebral palsy, or a variable combination of these conditions.

Other teratogenic organisms are those of toxoplasmosis and syphilis.

Drugs. The potential danger of new drugs was exemplified by the nonbarbiturate sedative, *thalidomide*. This drug was introduced in West Germany in the late 1950s and it was also marketed in other Western European countries. In 1959–1961 thousands of babies in West Germany and hundreds in other countries were born with partial or complete absence of the limbs, or with other defects. The mothers were found to have taken thalidomide early in pregnancy. A daily intake for one week was sufficient to induce limb defects. Before the drug was released, animal trials had given no grounds for suspicion. However, later tests showed that limb defects could in fact be induced in the offspring of pregnant rabbits and rats. The thalidomide disaster has led to extreme caution in the introduction of new drugs for commercial distribution, especially because irreparable harm may be done to the human embryo before the mother is known to be pregnant.

It might be thought that the antimitotic drugs used in cancer therapy would be especially harmful to the rapidly growing embryo. However, only *aminopterin*—a folic acid antagonist —has proved to be teratogenic in man. This substance has been used in order to bring about abortion. When it fails to induce abortion the offspring is likely to show multiple malformations.

None of the *hormones* has been clearly incriminated following administration to pregnant women. In mice and rabbits, cortisone is known to induce cleft palate in the offspring. Sporadic cases of cleft palate have been recorded in humans following the intake of cortisone, but their number has been insufficient to warrant withdrawal of the drug from patients requiring it.

Of the *antibiotics,* only the tetracyclines may give rise to an anomaly. When these drugs are administered during the period of enamel formation, they may produce yellowing of the deciduous teeth.

Epileptic mothers taking *anticonvulsant drugs, e.g.,* phenytoin, barbiturates, are about three times as likely as normal mothers, or epileptic mothers not taking drugs, to give birth to malformed babies.

The teratogenic action of lysergic acid diethylamide (LSD) is unproven. Several small series of studies have implicated LSD in the appearance of defects in the hands and feet of offspring whose mothers have taken this drug either before or during pregnancy.

There is some reason to believe that pregnant women working in operating theaters (anesthetists, operating nurses) have an increased risk of giving birth to malformed babies. The responsible factor could be one or more of the anesthetic gases.

Radiation. It is well known that the use of *roentgen rays,* or *radium,* in the treatment of pregnant patients having pelvic tumors is likely to produce skeletal abnormalities in the fetuses. The exposure of pregnant women to severe atomic radiation, as in the Hiroshima and Nagasaki explosions, led to a fetal–neonatal death rate of about 40%. The infants who survived tended to show evidence of brain-cell damage.

Irradiation of the gonads, even at very low levels (50r) may induce *mutation* of the germ cells—a sudden and permanent change in genetic structure, capable of transmitting congenital defects through subsequent generations.

Autoimmunization. Considerable interest was aroused by the observation that mothers of infants born without thyroid glands, *i.e.,* athyroid cretins, may have antithyroid antibodies in their blood. This observation suggests that products of embryonic organ primordia may cross the placenta, inducing maternal antibody production; the antibodies may return to the embryo and interfere with organ differentiation. Animal experiments do not indicate that a mechanism of this kind is common although anti-kidney antibodies injected into pregnant rats have yielded abnormalities including renal aplasia.

SUGGESTED READING

Goss RJ: Theories of growth regulation. In Regulation of Organ and Tissue Growth. New York, Academic Press, 1972, pp 1–12

Gruenwald P: Mechanisms of abnormal embryonic development. In de Alvarez RR (ed): Clinical Obstetrics and Gynecology. New York, Hoeber, 1966, pp 598–607

Hamburgh M: Theories of induction. In Barrington WSW, Willis AJ (eds): Theories of Differentiation. London, Arnold, 1971, pp 36–63

McKeown T, Record RG: Malformations in a population observed for five years after birth. In Wolstenholme GEW, O'Connor CM (eds): Ciba Foundation Symposium on Congenital Malformations. Boston, Little, Brown & Co, 1961, pp 2–16

Poswillo D: Mechanisms and pathogenesis of malformations. Br Med Bull 32:59–64, 1976

Tarin D: Tissue interactions in morphogenesis, morphostasis and carcinogenesis. J Theor Biol 34:61–72, 1972

Wilson JG: Principles of teratology. In Environment and Birth Defects. New York, Academic Press, 1973, pp 12–34

Chapter 2

gametogenesis

THE REPRODUCTIVE ORGANS

The human reproductive organs may be divided into primary and secondary structures. The primary sex organ, or *gonad*, is responsible for the production of the gametes. The secondary sex organs are responsible for the transport and nourishment of the gametes.

The *testis* is the male gonad, and the *spermatozoon* (or sperm) is its gamete. The ovary is the female gonad, and its gamete is the *ovum*. At fertilization, spermatozoon and ovum unite to form the zygote. The line of cells that gives rise to a gamete is known as the *germ plasm.* The cells that are not in direct line, and whose plasm, *i.e.,* nucleoplasm and cytoplasm, therefore dies with the individual, are called somatic cells, *i.e.,* body cells, as distinct from sex cells.

MALE REPRODUCTIVE ORGANS

The paired testes lie outside the abdominal cavity in the pouchlike scrotum. Fibrous septa subdivide the organ into about 300 lobes, and these are filled by the convoluted *seminiferous tubules* (Fig. 2-1). The spermatozoa are expressed from the seminiferous tubules into a network of ducts, the *rete testis;* from the rete they pass by *efferent ductules* to the *epididymis*. The head of the epididymis is made up of coiled efferent ductules; these unite to form a single duct whose convolutions form the body and tail of the epididymis. From the tail the *ductus (vas) deferens* runs up to enter the abdominal cavity through the inguinal canal. Descending to the pelvis it terminates by union with the duct of the *seminal vesicle.* The common channel so formed is the *ejaculatory duct,* and this pierces the *prostate* to enter the urethra. The ducts of the prostate and the small *bulbourethral glands* open directly into the urethra. The urethra is also part of the urinary system; it runs forward in the penis to open at the external urethral orifice.

FEMALE REPRODUCTIVE ORGANS

The female reproductive system is contained in the pelvis. The paired ovaries are attached to the back of the *broad ligament*—a peritoneal fold passing from the uterus to the side wall of the pelvis (Fig. 2-2). Running in the upper margin of the broad ligament is the

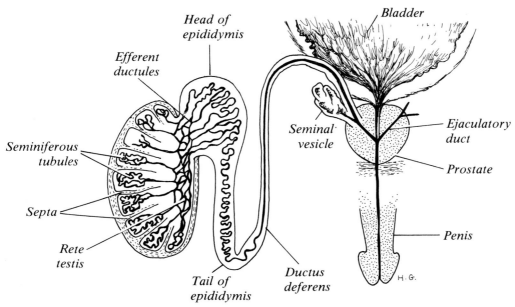

FIG. 2-1. Male reproductive organs.

FIG. 2-2. Female reproductive organs.

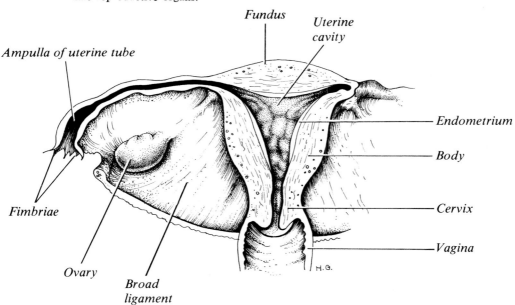

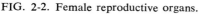

uterine tube, or *oviduct.* The lateral one-third of the tube is the expanded *ampulla,* and from the opening of the ampulla several fingerlike processes, the *fimbriae,* are directed towards the ovary. The medial end of the tube pierces the wall of the uterus and opens into its lumen. The lining mucous membrane of the tube is deeply folded and the epithelium is ciliated.

The uterus is a highly muscular organ occupying the middle of the pelvis. It comprises the *fundus,* located above the level of entry of the uterine tubes; a main part or *body;* and the neck, or *cervix,* which projects into the *vagina* below. The mucous membrane of the uterus is known as the *endometrium.* The vagina leads downward and forward from the cervix to open between the urethra in front and the anus behind.

DEVELOPMENT OF THE GAMETES

Gametogenesis is the development of the male and female germ cells from their precursors in the gonads. When the development of the gonads themselves comes to be considered, it will be seen that the remote precursors—the *primordial germ cells*—are set aside at an early stage in the history of the individual. However, we are concerned here with the immediate precursors found at puberty. The development of the spermatozoon and of the ovum will be considered in turn.

SPERMATOGENESIS

Each seminiferous tubule is tightly coiled within its testicular lobe. Outside the tubule the vascular connective tissue contains *interstitial,* or *Leydig,* cells. These cells secrete *testosterone,* the hormone that maintains the accessory sex organs (seminal vesicles, prostate, and bulbourethral glands).

Spermatogenesis takes place in the epithelium of the seminiferous tubules. Two processes are involved: 1) maturation, by which the primitive precursor gives rise to the highly specialized spermatozoon, and 2) a reduction of the chromosome complement of the gamete to one-half. The union of the male gamete with the female (similarly reduced) will restore the full chromosome count.

Two kinds of cells make contact with the lining basement membrane (Fig. 2-3). The first is the *spermatogonium.* The second is the long, supporting or *Sertoli cell,* which extends to the lumen of the tubule. The spermatogonium resembles the somatic cells of the male in having 46 chromosomes. This is the full, or *diploid,* number, made up of 22 pairs of autosomes and two nonidentical *sex chromosomes* (called X and Y). Like a somatic cell, the spermatogonium divides by mitosis, each chromosome splitting longitudinally so that 46 pass to each daughter cell. In this way a spermatogonium may give rise to 1) two new spermatogonia, or 2) cells that (after repeated mitosis) enlarge to form *primary spermatocytes.* The primary spermatocyte divides by meiosis. Each of the two *secondary spermatocytes* of the first division of meiosis has a *haploid* number (*haplos,* half) of chromosomes (22 + X, or 22 + Y), the chromosomes being double-stranded except at the centromere. The second division yields *spermatids,* each with a haploid number of single-stranded chromosomes. Electron microscopy has revealed intercellular bridges between the members of successive generations of cells, including the newly formed spermatids.

SPERMIOGENESIS

Many spermatids are incorporated in the free extremity of each Sertoli cell, and there they undergo a remarkable metamorphosis to become spermatozoa. The metamorphosis of the spermatid is known as *spermiogenesis.* The nucleus of the spermatid becomes progressively more compact and forms the *head* of the spermatozoon. The posterior of the two centrioles lengthens to form the *tail,* or *flagellum,* and the anterior centriole encircles the area between head and tail, at the *neck.* Vesicles from the Golgi zone form the *acrosome,* which covers the anterior part of the head. The middle piece (anterior half of tail) acquires a cuff of mitochondria. Redundant cytoplasm is shed, the mature sperm being enclosed by a thin film of cytoplasm within the cell membrane.

The fluid in the seminiferous tubules is thought to be secreted by Sertoli's cells. The sperm are carried passively by the fluid to the epididymis, where they are stored.

OOGENESIS

The ovary is composed of an outer *cortex* and an inner *medulla*. The cortex, in which the germ cells develop, has a richly cellular web, or *stroma*, of connective tissue in which the ovarian vessels ramify.

The homologue of the spermatogonium is the *oogonium*. Oogonia resembles the somatic cells of the female in having 22 pairs of autosomes and twin sex chromosomes (X and X). Like the spermatogonia, they divide by mitosis. Before birth, the offspring of the oogonia, will full chromosome complements, enlarge to become *primary oocytes*. Each one is surrounded by a layer of flat cells derived from the surface epithelium of the ovary (Fig. 2-4A), the oocyte and its epithelium forming an *ovarian follicle*.

Shortly before birth the primary oocytes enter the prophase of the first division of meiosis. For reasons unknown, meiosis proceeds no further until the onset of the ovarian cycle at puberty. However, the majority of the ovarian follicles degenerate early in postnatal life; of the 200,000 present at birth, only some 10,000 survive until puberty.

The development of an ovum, like that of a spermatozoon, entails the processes of maturation and chromosome reduction. It will be seen that the behavior of the chromosomes of maturing female gametes is identical to that of the male homologues. From what has been said, however, a fundamental *time* difference is apparent in the behavior of male and female

FIG. 2-3. Diagram of spermatogenesis.

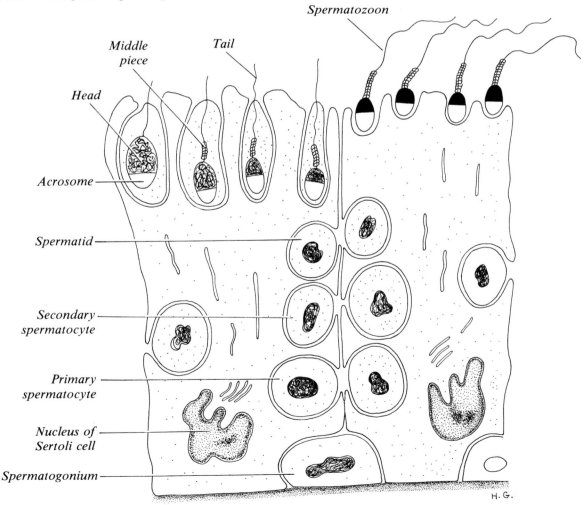

H. G.

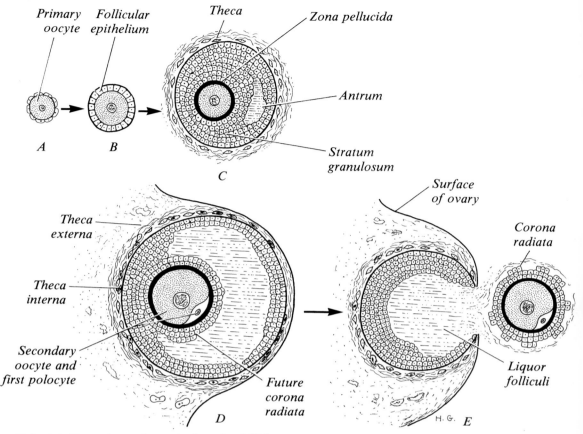

FIG. 2-4. Formation and growth of ovarian follicle.

stem cells. The spermatogonia multiply throughout reproductive life, producing a continuous succession of spermatocytes, whereas mitotic division of oogonia has already ceased before birth.

THE OVARIAN CYCLE

With the onset of sexual maturity the ovary and uterus undergo monthly cyclic changes. At the commencement of the ovarian cycle a crop of follicles begins the process of maturation (Fig. 2-4). As a rule only one follicle ripens fully; the remainder, numbering up to a hundred, atrophy after a variable period of growth.

The epithelial cells of enlarging follicles become columnar (Fig. 2-4B) and the adjacent stroma forms a concentric shell, or *theca,* around them; a basement membrane appears between follicle and theca, and a second, thick membrane—the *zona pellucida*—develops around the oocyte. With continued growth the follicular cells form the many-layered *stratum granulosum* (Fig. 2-4C). The electron microscope shows the zona pellucida to be amorphous. It is thought to be synthesized by Golgi complexes located beneath the plasma membrane of the oocyte (or *vitelline membrane*). The granulosa cells too are actively secretory, as indicated by well-developed Golgi complexes and endoplasmic reticulum. They project processes into the zona pellucida and many make contact with the vitelline membrane (Fig. 2-5). The membrane shows numerous microvilli and pinocytotic vesicles, indicating the absorption of metabolites passed to the oocyte by the granulosa cells.

A fluid-filled cavity, or *antrum,* appears in the stratum granulosum (Fig. 2-4C). With its appearance the follicle is called *vesicular,* or *graafian.* The thecal capsule itself is enlarging meanwhile, developing a fibromuscular *theca externa* and a *theca interna* whose large cells secrete estrogenic hormone and are called the *thecal gland.* Estrogenic hormone stimulates development of the endometrium. As the graafian follicle nears maturity the nucleus of the primary oocyte moves to the surface of the cell and completes meiotic division. Half the chromosomes $(22 + X)$ pass into each daughter cell. The division of the primary oocyte is very unequal, one daughter cell (*first polocyte,* or *first polar body*) being extruded with its chromosomes in a minute droplet of cytoplasm (Fig. 2-4D). (This tiny cell may subdivide but is of no functional importance.) The other cell is the *secondary oocyte.*

FIG. 2-5. Fine structural appearance of stratum granulosum, zona pellucida (ZP), and surface of oocyte. (From micrographs kindly supplied by Dr D. Szollosi.)

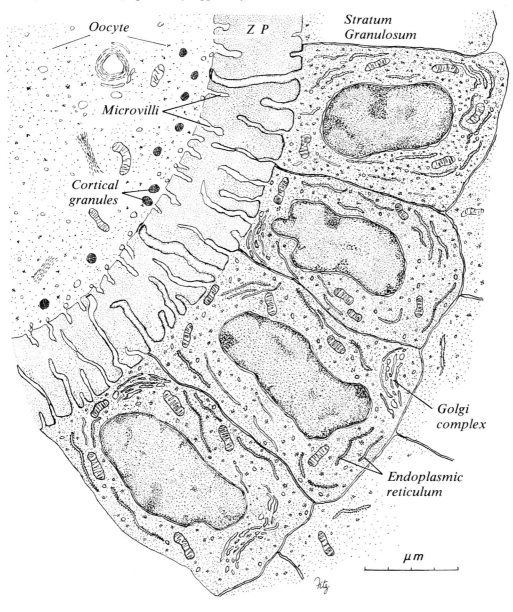

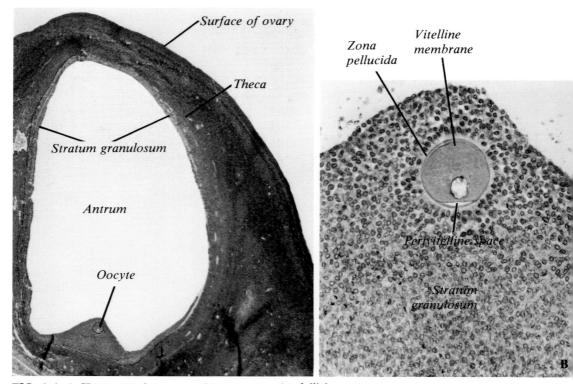

FIG. 2-6. **A.** Human ovarian cortex with mature ovarian follicle.
B. Enlargement from A.
(From a negative kindly supplied by Dr E. Roosen-Runge.) (**A,** x9; **B,** x60)

The single follicle that matures fully each month attains a final diameter of about 12 mm (Fig. 2-6). The contained *liquor folliculi* forms a blister at the surface of the ovary (Fig. 2-4D). Continued increase in the amount of liquor folliculi is followed by rupture (Fig. 2-4E), which may be assisted by contraction of smooth muscle in the theca externa. The secondary oocyte, now about 130 μm in diameter, is deposited with its investing granulosa cells at the mouth of the uterine tube. This event is termed *ovulation,* although the chromosomal changes leading to the formation of the definitive ovum are not yet complete. Upon its expulsion from the follicle the oocyte enters upon the second division of meiosis. This again is very unequal and gives rise to the ovum, on the other hand, and the *second polocyte* (*second polar body*) on the other. The second division is not completed, nor is the second polocyte extruded, unless fertilization takes place. Ovulation occurs 14 ± 2 days before the onset of the next menstrual cycle. Bleeding caused by tearing of the cortical blood vessels is trivial in amount, but it may suffice to irritate the parietal peritoneum of the lower abdominal wall, giving rise to *mittelschmerz* ("middle-pain," *i.e.,* pain at mid-cycle).

THE CORPUS LUTEUM

The interior of the ruptured follicles is filled with a coagulum derived from torn thecal capillaries (Fig. 2-7A). The granulosa cells enlarge and become tinged with a yellow pigment, and are now called *granulosa lutein cells.* Cells of the theca interna enlarge also, and are called *theca lutein cells.* Sinusoidal capillaries invade the luteal-cell mass to complete the *corpus luteum* by the fourth postovulatory day (Fig. 2-7B). The granulosa lutein cells secrete *progesterone,* which, together with estrogen secreted by the theca lutein cells is responsible for the premenstrual build-up of the endometrium. If the ovum is *not* fertilized the

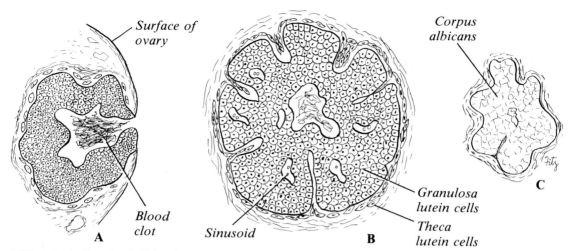

FIG. 2-7. **A.** Graafian follicle after rupture.
B. Corpus luteum.
C. Corpus albicans.

corpus luteum, after ten days, undergoes rapid regression and fibrosis to form a pale scar (the *corpus albicans*) in the ovarian cortex (Fig. 2-7C). Two weeks after liberation of the ovum the ovarian cycle is renewed in another crop of follicles. If the ovum *is* fertilized, and imbeds in the uterus, the corpus luteum persists and enlarges.

The ovarian cycle is regulated by the hormonal activities of the pituitary gland and hypothalamus. These functions are outside the scope of the present description.

THE UTERINE CYCLE

The endometrium of the body and fundus of the uterus displays a monthly cycle of growth, shedding, and renewal, referred to as the *uterine cycle,* or *menstrual cycle.* The cycle is in phase with the ovarian cycle and is regulated by ovarian hormones (Fig. 2-8). There are four phases:

The Proliferative or Estrogenic Phase

The proliferate phase lasts 10 ± 1 days. The endometrium is not completely shed each month; the basal portion, 0.5 mm thick, remains attached to the myometrium. This *basal layer* is essential for the renewal of the mucosa following menstruation or childbirth. It contains the stumps of the uterine glands, with vascular connective tissue (stroma) between. The epithelium is first restored by surface spread of cells from the gland stumps. Then, under the control of estrogenic hormone secreted by a crop of enlarging ovarian follicles, all the elements of the mucosa proliferate. The glands lengthen to 2 mm and the stromal cells and blood vessels multiply.

The Secretory or Progestational Phase

The secretory phase lasts 13 ± 1 days. When the ovum has been liberated and the corpus luteum begins to develop the endometrium is influenced both by granulosa luteal-cell progesterone and by theca luteal-cell estrogen. Droplets of glycogen-rich secretion appear in the uterine glands, which acquire a characteristic "saw-tooth" appearance in histologic sections. The arteries running between the glands are known as the *spiral arteries.* Three

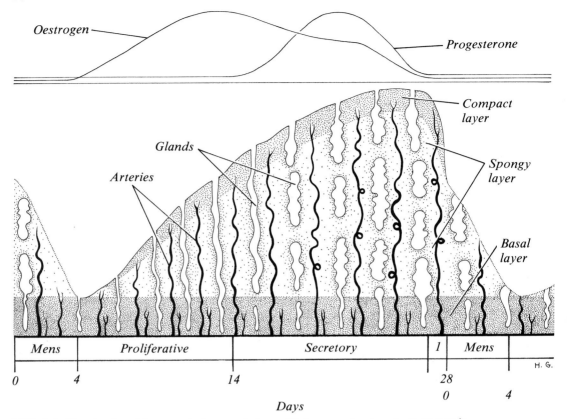

FIG. 2-8. Structural and hormonal changes during a 28-day menstrual cycle. I, Ischemic phase; Mens, Menstrual phase.

layers can now be recognized in the endometrium—a superficial, densely cellular *compact layer;* an intermediate *spongy layer,* packed with hypertrophic glands; and the *basal layer.* The compact and spongy layers become edematous, *i.e.,* rich in intercellular fluid, towards the end of this phase. The basal layer takes no part in the endometrial changes of the menstrual cycle or pregnancy; its function is to regenerate mucosa lost at menstruation or parturition.

If the ovum is fertilized the endometrium is now ready to receive it. If not, then the corpus luteum degenerates, the ovarian hormones are withdrawn, and menstruation follows.

The Ischemic Phase

The ischemic phase lasts one day. Hormone withdrawal leads to constriction of the spiral arteries with resultant ischemic necrosis of the compact and spongy layers. The intercellular fluid is resorbed and the endometrium shrinks to half its previous height. The spiral arteries then relax, and the returning blood flow dislodges the necrotic endometrium into the uterine lumen.

The Menstrual Phase

The menstrual phase lasts 4 ± 1 days. This is the phase of external bleeding, or menstruation. Hemorrhage in different areas of the uterus leads to a gradual shedding of all but the basal layer of the endometrium. Total blood loss amounts to 50–60 ml. The first day of a menstruation is regarded as the first day of the menstrual cycle, because 1) it is the most easily recognized stage, and 2) the maturation of a new crop of ovarian follicles commences on that day.

GERM CELL ABNORMALITIES

Some 10% of married couples suffer from *infertility, i.e.,* involuntary sterility. When the gynecologist is consulted his investigations are not restricted to the female partner. In at least one-third of cases the cause is to be looked for in the male. Among the possible causes of male infertility is defective sperm production, in which few or no live sperm are produced (*azoospermia*), or there is a high incidence of malformed sperm as revealed by examination of an ejaculate under the light microscope. Malformed sperm are considered significant only if their number exceeds 20% of the total sperm count on repeated examination. Sperm motility normally persists for more than six hours after seminal emission.

An ovum or spermatozoon of normal fertilizing capacity may contain an incorrect number of chromosomes. During meiosis the homologous chromosomes may not all separate evenly from the equatorial plate. A chromatid may pass to an incorrect daughter cell, yielding one gamete with 24 chromosomes and one with 22. When the error involves an autosome the zygote will have either three homologous chromosomes (two from one parent and one from the other)—a condition known as *trisomy*—or only one (*monosomy*). A similar fault may affect the sex chromosomes, and chromosome counts (*karyotypes*) with 44 + XXX, 44 + XXY, or 44 + XYY may be identified in the offspring. The leukocytes of the blood are used to obtain karyotypes, but all the cells of the body will contain the same abnormality. Many individuals with an extra chromosome display a physical appearance that is characteristic for the particular chromosome involved. The commonest is Down's syndrome (formerly called mongolism), in which there is an additional 21st autosome (trisomy 21). Down's syndrome is relatively frequent in the offspring of women over 40 years of age, indicating that the failure of separation (*nondisjunction*) has taken place in an oocyte of advanced age.

SUGGESTED READING

Biggers JD, Schuetz AW: Oogenesis. Baltimore, University Park Press, 1972

Courot M, de Riviers MH, Ortavant R: Spermatogenesis. In Johnson AD, Gomes WR, Vandemark NL (eds): The Testis, Vol 1. New York, Academic Press, 1970, pp. 339–432

Dym M, Fawcett DW: The blood–testis barrier in the rat and the physiological compartmentation of the seminiferous epithelium. Biol Reprod 3:308–320, 1970

Gamzell C: Ovulation. In Scientific Foundations of Obstetrics and Gynecology. London, Heinemann, 1970, pp 131–134

Hancock JL: The sperm cell. Science J 6:31–38, 1970

Kang Y: Development of the zona pellucida in the rat oocyte. Am J Anat 139:535–566, 1974

Chapter 3

fertilization and cleavage: the blastocyst

FERTILIZATION

During coitus the spermatozoa (sperm) are propelled to the male urethra by the smooth muscle of epididymis and ductus deferens. The secretions of the seminal vesicles, prostate, and bulbourethral glands are added to the spermatozoa. The aggregate mass is the *semen,* or seminal fluid, which contains about 100 million spermatozoa per milliliter. At the male climax, when ejaculation takes place, 3–5 ml of semen are deposited high in the vagina.

The spermatozoa are motile within the semen. In the seminiferous tubules and epididymis they are nonmotile. It has been found experimentally that spermatozoa from the epididymis become motile when the epididymal secretion is washed from them. The seminal fluid may confer motility by dilution of an epididymal inhibitory factor.

On encountering the watery, alkaline mucous secretion of the cervix, the spermatozoa swim upward through it. Their passage is assisted by the hydrolysis of cervical mucus by seminal protease enzymes. When they reach the internal os their further ascent is brought about by gentle contractions of the uterus and uterine tubes. These movements carry them to the outer part of the uterine tube within six hours of coitus.

The great majority of the spermatozoa survive for less than 24 hours in the female genital tract. However, there is reason to believe that an occasional one may be able to fertilize an oocyte as long as three days after coitus.

Sperm taken directly from an ejaculate, and introduced to an oocyte in the uterine tube, are incapable of fertilizing the oocyte. They must first be *capacitated, i.e.,* given the capacity to fertilize, by passage through the uterus. The nature of capacitation is unknown; it does not alter the appearance of the sperm. It may be that a protective coating is removed by uterine secretions.

The secondary oocyte is capable of being fertilized for a period of 24 hours (or less) after ovulation. When liberated from the ovary it is surrounded by the zona pellucida and by 3000–4000 cells of the stratum granulosum. The granulosa cells assume a radial disposition and are known as the *corona radiata.* The entire cell mass is grasped by the fimbriae of the free end of the uterine tube. Entry into the tube is effected by the cilia of the fimbrial epithelium. Fertilization usually takes place in the tubal ampulla.

Of the millions of spermatozoa contained in the ejaculate, only a few thousand appear to enter the uterine tubes, and only a few hundred reach the vicinity of the ovum. This small number is, of course, more than sufficient since only one sperm will impregnate the ovum.

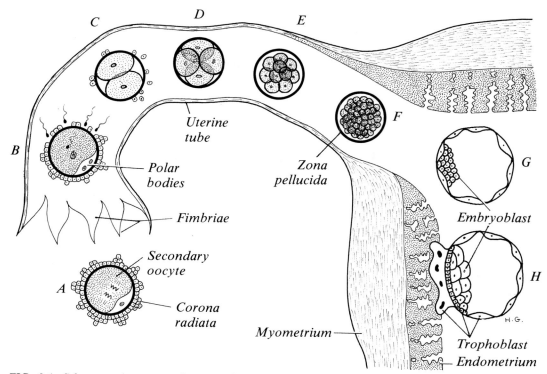

FIG. 3-1. Scheme to show successive stages from ovulation to the commencement of implantation.

FIG. 3-2. Living human oocyte and spermatozoa photographed on a slide. (Reproduced by permission of Dr L. B. Shettles and Urban and Schwarzenberg.) (x400)

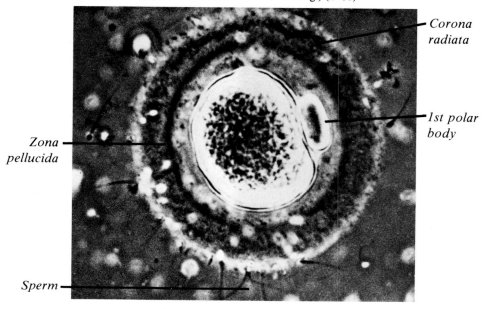

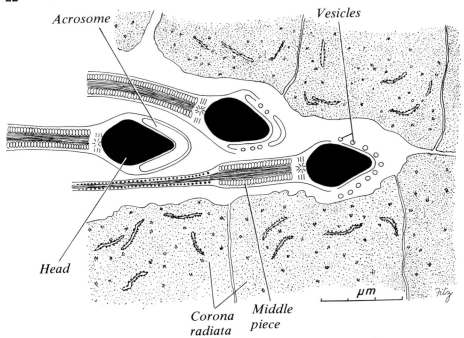

Acrosome

Vesicles

Head

Corona radiata *Middle piece*

μm

FIG. 3-3. Acrosomal changes during sperm penetration of the corona radiata.

Many spermatozoa penetrate among the cells of the corona radiata (Figs. 3-1 and 3-2). As they enter the corona they display the *acrosome reaction,* in which the outer membrane of the acrosome fuses at intervals with the plasma membrane investing the heads of the sperm (Fig. 3-3). *Between* the vesicles created in this way, the contents of the acrosome are liberated. The acrosome is the richest known source of the enzyme *hyaluronidase,* and it is thought that sperm penetration of the corona is aided by solvent action of hyaluronidase on glycosaminoglycans in its intercellular cement. In addition, proteolytic enzymes contained in the acrosome may facilitate the passage of sperm through the zona pellucida.

The corona radiata persists until fertilization has taken place; whereupon the corona cells begin to die, and as they do so they separate from the zona pellucida, and from one another.

Many sperm pierce the zona pellucida and enter the perivitelline space. Only one sperm penetrates the vitelline membrane. The mode of penetration by the human spermatozoon is unknown. In laboratory mammals at least, the spermatozoon makes tangential contact. The plasma membrane covering the posterior part of the head breaks down, as does the underlying vitelline membrane. The ooplasm engulfs the entire spermatozoon. The neck and tail of the spermatozoon detach from the head, and disintegrate. The head itself undergoes decondensation, enlarging and revealing its nucleoprotein strands. It is called the *male pronucleus.*

The mechanism by which only one spermatozoon penetrates the vitelline membrane is uncertain. In laboratory mammals, *cortical granules* (Fig. 2-5) appear deep to the vitelline membrane immediately after ovulation. The granules persist until one spermatozoon pierces the vitelline membrane; then their contents are liberated by exocytosis into the perivitelline space. It is reasonable to believe that this *cortical reaction* is concerned in preventing the entry of further sperm.

Penetration of the vitelline membrane triggers completion of the second reduction division in the oocyte. The second polocyte is extruded into the perivitelline space (Fig. 3-1B). The nucleus of the definitive *ovum* is called the *female pronucleus.*

The male and female pronuclei approach one another and join. Their chromatin strands intermingle, the diploid number of chromosomes is restored, and the zygote is complete. The chromosomal constitution of the female pronucleus is 22 + X. Union with a male pronucleus of constitution 22 + X will yield a female zygote (44 + XX); union with a male pronucleus of constitution 22 + Y will yield a male zygote (44 + XY).

The zygote measures less than 0.2 mm in diameter. Although it is the largest cell in the body, it is scarcely visible to the naked eye. It is a seemingly simple cell with no dramatic ultrastructural features, but at the molecular level it is by far the most sophisticated of all biological systems. Sustained by the metabolites it finds in the genital tract, it multiplies prodigiously to yield the countless millions of cells that make up the tissues, organs, and body systems of postnatal anatomy—in a word, it is *totipotent*. Its genetic constitution will ensure that the individual is not alone human, but unique—from the pattern of the fingerprints to the number, color, shape, and length of the eyelashes.

Within two weeks of fertilization one or more daughter cells are segregated in the wall of the nourishing yolk sac. These are the progenitor cells of the next human generation. The moment of fertilization, therefore, is the culmination and climax of events that have been set in train twenty or more years previously. The pregnant mother carries not only her child but a parent of her grandchild as well.*

CLEAVAGE

Cleavage, or *segmentation,* is the phase of repeated cell division that transforms the zygote into a morula. It begins on the day following fertilization. During the period of cleavage, which lasts about four days, the dividing cells are contained by the zona pellucida. As they increase in number they therefore become progressively smaller (Fig. 3-1C–F). At the same time the cilia lining the uterine tube thrust the dividing zygote towards the uterus.

At the first cleavage the zygote enters into mitotic division. The chromosomes split in the usual way and the two daughter cells receive equal numbers of maternal and paternal chromosomes.

At the second cleavage, each daughter cell divides. Further segmentation produces 4-cell, 8-cell, and 16-cell stages. The period of the morula extends from the 16-cell stage until blastocyst formation commences when the cluster of cells numbers 50–60.

THE BLASTOCYST

The morula enters the uterus on the fourth or fifth day after fertilization. During the following one or two days it lies free in the uterine lumen, bathed by the secretion of the uterine glands. The zona pellucida is dissolved and a fluid-filled cavity appears within the morula, which is then known as a *blastocyst* (Fig. 3-1G). The shell of the blastocyst is composed of the flat-celled trophoblast. Inside, against one pole, is the round-celled embryoblast.

---

* The concept of the succession of generations was put in literary form by James Joyce, in *Ulysses:*
"To reflect that each one who enters imagines himself to be the first to enter whereas he is always the last term of a preceding series even if the first term of a succeeding one, each imagining himself to be first, last, only and alone, whereas he is neither first nor last nor only nor alone in a series originating in and repeated to infinity."

SUGGESTED READING

Biggers JD, Borland RM: Physiological aspects of growth and development of the preimplantation mammalian embryo. Ann Rev Physiol 38:95–119, 1976

Dukelow WR, Riegle GD: Transport of gametes and survival of the ovum as function of the oviduct. In Johnson AD, Foley GW (eds): The Oviduct and Its Functions. New York, Academic Press, 1974, pp 193–220

Edwards RG: Advances in reproductive biology and their implication for studies on human congenital defects. In Motulsky AG, Lenz W (eds): Birth Defects. Amsterdam, Excerpta Medica Int Congr Ser No. 310, 1974, pp 92–104

Hertig AT, Adams EC, Mulligan WJ: On the preimplantation stages of the human ovum. A description of four normal and four abnormal specimens ranging from the second to the fifth day of development. Contrib Embryol Carnegie Inst 35:199–220, 1954

Shettles LB: Ovum Humanum. New York, Hafner, 1960

Soupart P: Fine morphology and physiology of the human fertilization process. In Campos da Paz A, Drill VA, Hayashi M, Rodrigues W, Schally AV (eds): Recent Advances in Human Reproduction. Amsterdam, Excerpta Medica, Int Congr Ser No. 370, 1975, pp 281–284

Chapter 4

implantation

On the sixth or seventh day after fertilization the blastocyst implants in the endometrium. In about two-thirds of cases it implants in the posterior wall of the body of the uterus; in about one-third it implants in the anterior wall.

Henceforth the development of the embryoblast and the trophoblast will proceed simultaneously. However, for descriptive purposes the two must be considered separately. It is sufficient here to state that, as the blastocyst implants, embryoblast and trophoblast cooperate to form two contiguous vesicles within the blastocyst. They are the *amniotic sac* and the *yolk sac.* A loose network of cells delaminates, *i.e.,* splits off, from the inner surface of the trophoblast. This is the *extraembryonic mesoderm;* it comes to line the inner surface of the trophoblast and the outer surface of the two vesicles (Fig. 4-1).

The trophoblast and its lining mesoderm are together known as the chorion.

The early differentiation of the chorion is summarized in Figure 4-1. Six stages are shown:

a. At the area of contact with the endometrium the flat trophoblastic cells become cuboidal, then multiply to form an outer syncytial layer, the *syncytiotrophoblast,* which invades the endometrium. The inner, cuboidal cells constitute the *cytotrophoblast.* Mitotic figures are abundant in the cytotrophoblast; disintegration of its plasma membranes can be observed with the electron microscope as new syncytium is formed from them.

b. Tongues of syncytiotrophoblast meet one another to enclose spaces, or *lacunae,* which initially contain endometrial tissue fluid. The endometrial sinusoids are soon eroded by the trophoblast, and their contents spill into the lacunae.

c. The proliferating cytotrophoblast enters the syncytial processes, forming cell columns (TC) within them. Thus are formed the *primary villi* of the placenta. These villi are not truly villous in form, however, as they interconnect freely.

d. The cytotrophoblastic cell columns push radially through the syncytium, then mushroom to unite with their neighbors and to create the *cytotrophoblastic shell* (CS), which surrounds the entire conceptus. The shell is pierced by maternal sinusoids at their points of rupture into the lacunae. The lacunae intercommunicate freely, giving rise to the labyrinthine *intervillous space.*

The extraembryonic mesoderm enters the villi, transforming them into *secondary villi.* It does not penetrate as far as the cytotrophoblastic shell.

e. Capillaries develop *in situ* from the extraembryonic mesoderm. Villi containing these blood vessels are called *tertiary.*

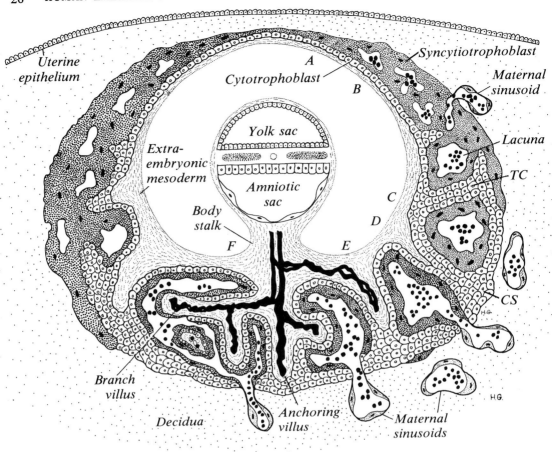

FIG. 4-1. Scheme to show early stages of implantation. TC, trophoblastic cell column; CS, cytotrophoblastic shell. Uterine glands are not represented in Figures 4-1 to 4-5.

f. *Anchoring villi* are those that gave rise to the trophoblastic shell. *Branch villi* sprout from their sides and float freely in the intervillous space.

The trophoblast, with its inner lining of extraembryonic mesoderm, forms the *chorionic vesicle (chorionic sac)*.

THE DECIDUAL REACTION

At the commencement of embedding the endometrium undergoes the *decidual reaction*, which begins at the implantation site and spreads throughout the endometrium in a few days. The stromal connective tissue cells enlarge greatly and are filled with glycogen and lipid. These *decidual cells* are readily seen in superficial curettings taken anywhere from the endometrium, and are diagnostic of pregnancy. Following the decidual reaction the endometrium is called the *decidua* throughout the remainder of the pregnancy.

The function of the decidual reaction is uncertain, but it appears to be more than nutritional. There is reason to believe that its main function is to counterbalance the invasive proclivity of the trophoblast. In mice, for example, the decidual reaction may be prevented by ovariectomy; transplantation of mouse trophoblast to this nonreactive mucous membrane results in the destruction of the underlying myometrium by deeply penetrating trophoblastic processes.

STAGES OF IMPLANTATION

Individual stages of implantation are represented in Figures 4-2 to 4-5. Figure 4-2A represents an ovum on the first day of implantation (approximately the seventh day after fertilization). The blastocyst always implants at its embryonic pole, *i.e.,* where embryoblast meets trophoblast. The flat-celled trophoblast lining the blastocyst has given rise to the cytotrophoblast, and this in turn to the syncytiotrophoblast. Deep to this the maternal capillaries have enlarged and multiplied. It is convenient to remember that the ovum begins to embed roughly one week after fertilization, and is completely embedded after another week.

Figure 4-2B represents the second day of implantation. The syncytiotrophoblast has commenced the erosion of maternal sinusoids by digestion of their endothelial lining. The cytotrophoblast has become many-layered.

Figure 4-3 shows the appearances on the 12th day after fertilization or 6th day of implantation. The amniotic sac and yolk sac have appeared, and the extraembryonic mesoderm has developed from the trophoblast. Embedding is nearly complete. The syncytiotrophoblast has formed lacunae, having tapped the material sinusoids. Within the lacunae the maternal blood is in direct contact with the trophoblast, the sinusoidal endothelium having been eroded.

Invasion of the uterine glands permits their secretion to be utilized for nutrition. Hemorrhage into eroded glands may find its way to the surface and give rise to a little external bleeding about ten days after implantation commences, *i.e.,* at the time of the next expected menstruation. The discharge of blood from the uterus may simulate menstruation and cause an error in calculating the date of delivery of the fetus from the menstrual history.

At 14 days or eighth day of implantation (Fig. 4-4) the syncytiotrophoblast is spreading radially on all sides, and the intervillous space is enlarging by the coalescence of lacunae. Cytotrophoblastic columns are also growing outwards, and secondary villi are forming by the extension of mesoderm into the columns.

At 16 days or tenth day of implantation (Fig. 4-5) the cytotrophoblastic shell is well developed. It is punctured by the maternal sinusoids. Blood vessels are differentiating from the chorionic mesoderm (Fig. 4-6); they will extend into the villi and into the mesodermal *body stalk,* which connects the chorion to the embryo.

FIG. 4-2. Implantation: **A**, first day; **B**, second day. (Adapted from Hertig AT, Rock J, Adams EC: Am J Anat 98:435–493, 1956)

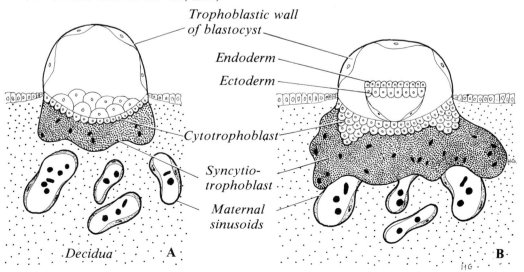

Trophoblastic wall
of blastocyst

Endoderm

Ectoderm

Cytotrophoblast

Syncytio-
trophoblast

Maternal
sinusoids

Decidua   **A**   **B**

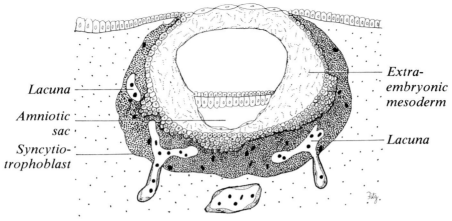

FIG. 4-3. Fifth day of implantation. (Adapted from Hertig AT, Rock J, Adams EC: Am J Anat 98:435–493, 1956)

FIG. 4-4. Eighth day of implantation. AS, amniotic sac; EEM, extraembryonic mesoderm; YS, yolk sac. (Adapted from Hertig AT, Rock J, Adams EC: Am J Anat 98:435–493, 1956)

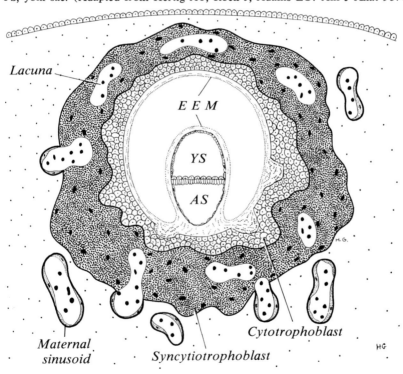

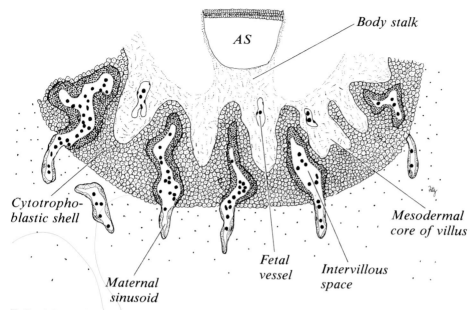

FIG. 4-5. Implantation, tenth day. AS, amniotic sac. (Adapted from Hertig AT, Rock J, Adams EC: Am J Anat 98:435–493, 1956)

FIG. 4-6. Part of the chorion on sixteenth day after fertilization. The field is comparable to the lower right part of Figure 4-5. Some of the maternal blood was hemolysed before or during fixation. Fetal vessels have not yet appeared in the villi. (Carnegie Collection) (x200)

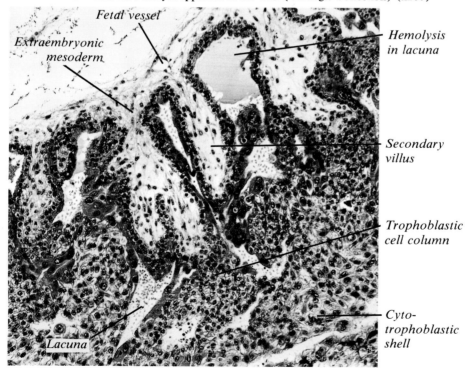

RELATIONSHIP OF FETAL TO MATERNAL BLOOD

The tertiary villi increase in complexity by means of side branches (Fig. 4-7A). Up to 200 treelike colonies of villi are formed, each fed by one fetal artery and drained by one fetal vein. Fetal and maternal blood are separated by the fetal capillary endothelium and by the trophoblast (Fig. 4-7B).

A sluggish circulation of maternal blood takes place through the early lacunae. The circulation becomes more brisk as the intervillous space enlarges. Fetal–maternal interchange is established during the fourth week with the establishment of the fetal circulation.

ENLARGEMENT OF THE CHORIONIC VESICLE

During the third week after fertilization the growing chorionic vesicle enlarges into the cavity of the uterus. The decidua outside the vesicle is now called the *decidua capsularis,* and that on the maternal aspect of the vesicle is the *decidua basalis* (Fig. 4-8A). The *decidua parietalis* lines the remainder of the body of the uterus. (The cervical mucous membrane does not undergo decidual change; it secretes a mucous plug that seals the cervical canal). After some 12 weeks of development the decidua capsularis comes into contact, and

FIG. 4-7. **A.** Tertiary chorionic villi during the fifth week after fertilization. The blood has been washed out of the intervillous space. (Cambridge Collection) (x150)
B. Field from section comparable to that shown in Figure 4-7A, enlarged. The intervillous space contains maternal blood. (Cambridge Collection) (x900)

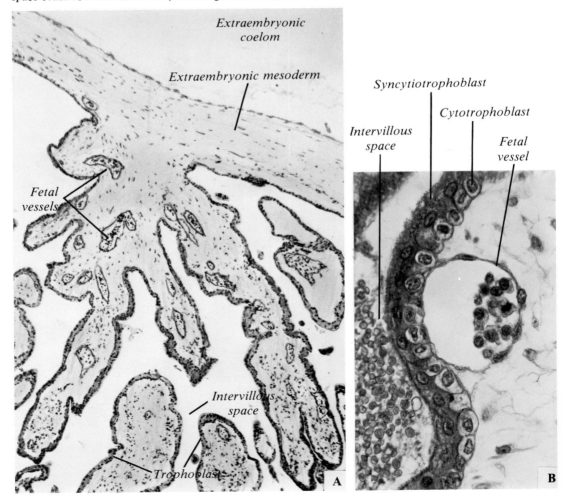

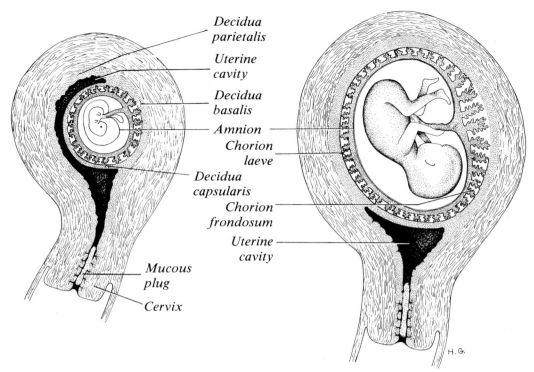

FIG. 4-8. Diagrams to illustrate enlargement of the chorionic vesicle and progressive obliteration of the uterine cavity. **A,** 6 weeks after fertilization; **B,** 16 weeks.

begins to fuse, with the decidua parietalis opposite (Fig. 4-8B). In this way the uterine cavity is gradually obliterated. Although the chorionic villi develop all around the blastocyst at first, the later (tertiary) villi become progressively restricted to the decidua basalis, where they enlarge to form the *chorion frondosum.* The *chorion laeve,* in contact with the thin decidua capsularis, undergoes atrophy.

The structure and functions of the mature placenta are considered in Chapter 13.

AN IMMUNOLOGIC RIDDLE

Tissues suitably transplanted from one region of an individual to another region survive and grow. Tissues donated by one individual to another genetically alien (allogeneic) to those of the host, are recognized as such by cells of the lymphoid series, and evoke an immune response which leads to their necrosis and rejection.

The conceptus has paternal genetic characters which differ from those of the mother. It should therefore be rejected shortly after implantation; yet it is not. The absence of the normal full-immune response on the part of the mother is one of the most provocative puzzles in immunology.

That the early embryo is itself antigenic can be shown by animal experiment; allogeneic embryonic tissues do not survive when implanted directly into host endometrium. The secret does not seem to lie in the decidual reaction associated with normal trophoblastic invasion because an extrauterine implantation site may support a pregnancy without showing any decidual reaction.

Evidently the trophoblast is responsible. That trophoblast cells are only weakly antigenic can be demonstrated experimentally by implanting them beneath the capsule of the kidney of an animal of the same strain, *i.e.,* as homografts. They survive well, even though they make intimate contact with the tissues of the host. Embryonic cells from the same conceptus are promptly rejected. In the normal course of implantation the human endometrium is locally infiltrated by leukocytes in a manner suggestive of a mild hypersensitivity reaction. The associated tissue tension (edema) may compress the endometrial lymphatics and interfere with access of paternally derived antigens to the regional lymph nodes. Alternatively, a chemical barrier may exist between trophoblast and endometrium; this barrier could reside in the *fibinoid substance* that appears on the maternal surface of the trophoblast.

ABNORMALITIES

ECTOPIC GESTATION

Ectopic gestation follows implantation of the ovum outside the uterine cavity. *Tubal gestation* is the most common form; it may result from failure of normal transport of the ovum because of disease of the uterine tube, or because ectopic endometrial tissue has developed in the tubal mucosa. Delayed ovulation may also be significant; should the ovum be fertilized towards the end of a menstrual cycle, reflux of maternal blood into the uterine tube at the onset of menstruation may encourage the blastocyst to implant there.

Whatever its cause, a tubal gestation becomes a grave surgical emergency during the second month following implantation. Rupture of the tube leads to severe intraperitoneal hemorrhage. Rarely the penetrating trophoblast may gain attachment to an abdominal organ, setting up a *secondary abdominal gestation.*

An *ovarian gestation* is one in which the oocyte is fertilized at the mouth of its ovarian follicle, and cleavage proceeds *in situ.* In a *primary abdominal gestation* the ovum implants (perhaps in ectopic endometrial tissue) on the peritoneal surface of an abdominal or pelvic organ, or on the abdominal wall. A functional placenta may develop, and a viable fetus has on occasion been delivered by cesarean section.

HYDATIDIFORM MOLE

Hydatidiform mole occurs in about 1% of pregnancies. It is characterized by cystic swelling of the chorionic mesoderm. The villi form grapelike clusters which may fill the uterine cavity. A fetus is usually absent.

CHORIOCARCINOMA

Choriocarcinoma is a very rare, highly malignant cancer derived from chorionic epithelium. It develops after the termination of pregnancy. For reasons unknown, islands of trophoblast retained within the uterus undergo sudden malignant change, invading the myometrium and uterine blood vessels.

SUGGESTED READING

Beer AE, Billingham RE, Scott JR: Immunogenetic aspects of implantation, placentation and feto-placental growth rates. Biol Reprod 12:176–189, 1975

Bøe F: Studies on the human placenta. III. Vascularization of the young foetal placenta. Vascularization of the chorionic villus. Acta Obstet Gynecol Scand 48:159–166, 1969

Enders AC: Anatomical aspects of implantation. J Reprod Fertil [Suppl] 25:1–15, 1976

Hamilton WJ, Boyd JD: Development of the human placenta. In Philipp E, Barnes J, Newton M (eds): Scientific Foundations of Obstetrics and Gynecology. London, Heinemann, 1970, pp 185–254

Hertig AT, Rock J, Adams EC: A description of 34 human ova within the first seventeen days of development. Am J Anat 98:435–493, 1956

Poland PJ, Dill FJ, Murray GJ: Embryonic development in ectopic human pregnancy. Teratology 14:315–321, 1976

Chapter 5

the germ layers and fetal membranes

BILAMINAR EMBRYONIC DISK

As implantation commences the embryoblast (Fig. 5-1A) begins to differentiate. It resolves into two apposed, disk-shaped cell layers, the *ectoderm* and the *endoderm*. The ectoderm is composed of columnar cells, the endoderm of cuboidal cells (Fig. 5-1B). Together the ectoderm and the endoderm give rise to the entire embryo, and they constitute the *bilaminar embryonic disk*.

AMNIOTIC SAC AND YOLK SAC

As the blastocyst sinks into the decidua the trophoblast forms a layer of flat cells, the *amnion* which attaches itself around the margin of the ectodermal disk (Fig. 5-1B). The cavity enclosed by amnion and ectoderm is the *amniotic sac*.

A few days later the extraembryonic mesoderm delaminates from the whole of the inner surface of the trophoblast (Fig. 5-1C). It forms a temporary membrane attached to the margin of the endoderm (Fig. 4-3). The *yolk sac* is created by the migration of endodermal cells along the inner surface of the membrane (Fig. 5-2A **arrows**).

EXTRAEMBRYONIC COELOM

Fluid-filled loculi in the extraembryonic mesoderm coalesce to form a new cavity, the *extraembryonic coelom,* which cleaves the mesoderm into visceral and parietal layers. The visceral layer surrounds the amniotic sac and yolk sac but it does not pass between them (Fig. 5-2). The parietal layer lines the interior of the trophoblast. It has already been noted that the parietal layer completes the chorion, and that it subsequently forms the connective tissue and blood vessels of the tertiary chorionic villi. Visceral and parietal layers are in broad continuity above the amniotic sac.

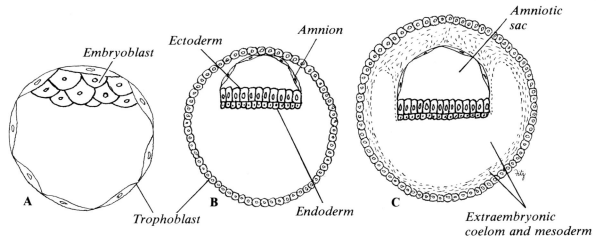

FIG. 5-1. Early differentiation of the blastocyst.

FIG. 5-2. Differentiation of the blastocyst (continued). **A.** Before the appearance of the embryonic axis.
B. After the axis has been defined by the prochordal plate. This is therefore a sagittal section viewed from the left side. EEM, extraembryonic mesoderm.

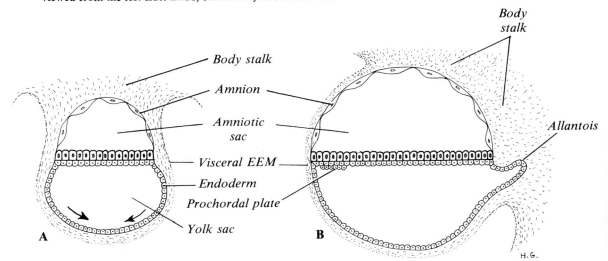

EMBRYONIC AXIS

A localized increase of the endoderm, called the *prochordal plate,* designates the future cephalic (rostral) end of the embryo (Fig. 5-2B). This plate is called prochordal because it later lies in front of *i.e.,* cranial to, the notochord. The embryo can now be described as having an *axis,* or orientation, with discernible rostral and caudal ends and left and right sides.

BODY STALK AND ALLANTOIS

The junctional region between the visceral and parietal portions of the extraembryonic mesoderm is the *body stalk.* It lies above the amnion at first (Fig. 5-2A), but soon shifts towards the caudal (tail) end of the embryo (Fig. 5-2B). It forms the only physical connection between embryo and placenta, and is the precursor of the *umiblical cord.*

The *allantois* is a narrow diverticulum that grows into the body stalk from the caudal part of the yolk sac (Fig. 5-2B). In many mammals the allantois invades the chorion and plays an important part in the development of the placenta—but one example of the variety of ways in which mammalian embryos make successful contact with the maternal bed. In man the allantois is vestigial and it does not reach the chorion.

The embryo represented by Figure 5-2B is two weeks old (from the date of fertilization). It is composed of the *embryo proper,* made up of the embryonic disk; and the *fetal membranes,* comprising the amnion, yolk sac, allantois, and chorion. The membranes are always referred to as "fetal," even in the embryonic period.

EMBRYONIC MESODERM

Ectodermal cells migrate to the midline on the 15th–16th day and form the *primitive streak.* The cells of the primitive streak migrate towards the roof of the underlying sac, then spread outward between ectoderm and endoderm. This intermediate layer is the *embryonic* (or intraembryonic) *mesoderm.*

In order to illustrate the development of the embryonic mesoderm, the amniotic sac in Figure 5-3A is being removed (in direction of arrow), leaving the primitive streak behind. The primitive streak is shown resting on the upper surface of the yolk sac. In Figure 5-3B the lower drawing represents the same view of the primitive streak and yolk sac. The *upper* drawing represents a median section in which the ectoderm is in place, the amnion being attached to its margins.

At its rostral end the primitive streak shows a thickening called the *primitive (Hensen's) node,* which displays a central *primitive pit.* From the primitive node a rod of cells grows rostrally beneath the ectoderm, as far as the posterior edge of the prochordal plate. This is the *notochordal process,* and from the primitive pit a narrow *notochordal canal* extends along its length.

FIG. 5-3. **A.** Schematic removal of amnion and ectoderm to show the spread of mesoderm (**B,** lower) from the primitive streak.
B, upper. The ectoderm is in place; the notochordal canal is not shown.

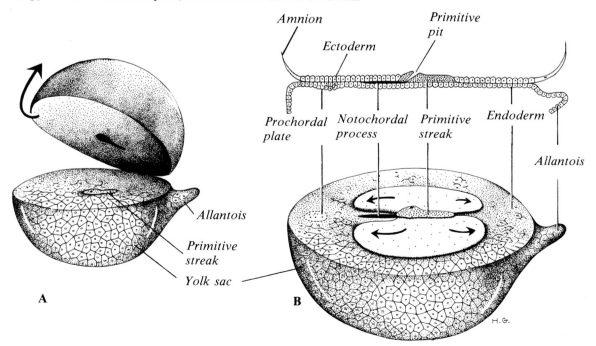

The embryonic mesoderm migrates outwards (**arrows** in Fig. 5-3B) and merges all around with the extraembryonic mesoderm. But at the prochordal plate, and immediately caudal to the primitive streak, ectoderm and endoderm remain in contact, no mesoderm intervening. These two areas are designated the *oral membrane* and the *cloacal membrane,* respectively. The mesoderm skirts these membranes (**arrows** in Fig. 5-4A) and reaches the midline at each end of the embryonic disk. Rostral to the oral membrane, it may be termed the *rostral mesoderm,* and caudal to the cloacal membrane, the *caudal mesoderm* (Fig. 5-4B). These two terms are coined here for purposes of description. The rostral mesoderm is taken to comprise the mesoderm beside, and rostral to, the oral membrane. It is usually referred to, *ab initio,* as the *cardiogenic mesoderm*—a misleading term, for it yields not only the cardiogenic crescent (from which the heart is derived), but also the septum transversum (which forms the connective tissue of the diaphragm and liver). The caudal mesoderm is taken to comprise the mesoderm beside, and caudal to, the cloacal membrane. It is usually unnamed until it gives rise to the genital tubercle during the formation of the embryonic tailfold. However, the caudal mesoderm also contributes to the lower part of the abdominal wall.

As the migration of cells from the primitive streak and node continues, the streak and node are progressively displaced in a caudal direction. The more rostral mesoderm, formed early in the third week, undergoes further development while new mesoderm continues to arise from the streak at the tail end of the embryo for a further week.

NOTOCHORD

The notochord is formed after temporary fusion of the notochordal process with the endoderm. First, the notochordal canal breaks through into the yolk sac cavity and the notochordal process is incorporated into the roof of the yolk sac (Fig. 5-4). In this way the notochordal canal is lost, and the opening into it from the primitive pit communicates directly with the yolk sac. The new passage is the *neurenteric canal.* Early in the third week the notochordal process rises up from the yolk sac and takes the form of a solid rod of cells —the *notochord.* With the formation of the notochord the neurenteric canal is obliterated.

FIG. 5-4. Continued development of the embryonic mesoderm. The extraembryonic mesoderm is not represented in this figure or in Figure 5-3.

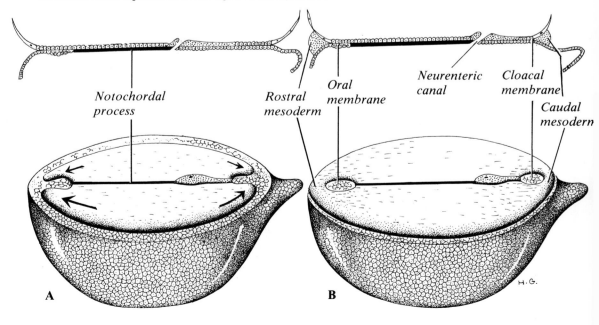

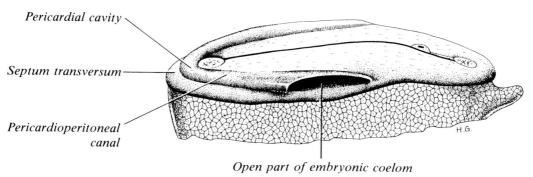

FIG. 5-5. The embryonic coelom.

FIG. 5-6. Transverse sections through the middle part of the embryonic coelom. In **A**, endoderm and embryonic mesoderm are shown; in **B**, ectoderm and amnion are also in place.

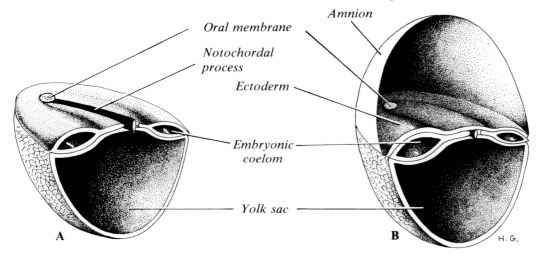

Appreciation of the significance of the behavior of the notochordal process requires an understanding of comparative chordate embryology.

The embryonic disk is now *trilaminar*. Its middle, mesodermal layer is deficient at the oral and cloacal membranes and also where the notochord occupies the midline.

EMBRYONIC COELOM

Fluid-filled spaces appear in the rostral mesoderm and in the outer part of the mesoderm at each side of the embryonic disk. The spaces coalesce to form the U-shaped *embryonic* (or intraembryonic) *coelom*. Opposite the middle two-thirds of the disk the coelom ruptures outwards to communicate with the extraembryonic coelom (Fig. 5-5).

The embryonic coelom is the precursor of the serous cavities. Its rostral part, straddling the midline, is the *pericardial cavity*. From it, paired *pericardioperitoneal canals* lead to the opening into the extraembryonic coelom. The mesoderm rostral to the pericardial cavity is the *septum transversum*.

Figure 5-6A represents a transverse section through the pericardioperitoneal canals shown in Figure 5-5. In Figure 5-6B the ectoderm and amnion have been restored.

SUGGESTED READING

Hamilton WJ, Mossman HW: Fertilization, cleavage and formation of the germ layers. In Hamilton, Boyd and Mossman's Human Embryology. Cambridge, Heffer, 1972, pp 54–82

Chapter 6

flexion of the embryo

As the embryo continues to grow it accommodates itself in the chorionic vesicle by folding. The process of folding, or *flexion,* begins at the margins of the embryonic disk. It is essential to bear in mind that flexion takes place all around the disk, so that the disk becomes dome-shaped. It is essential also to realize that, while flexion is taking place, growth and differentiation continue. The most significant events occurring *pari passu* are these: 1) early development of the nervous system; 2) segmentation of the mesoderm; 3) the appearance of the branchial arches; and 4) foundation of the cardiovascular system. An appreciation of the first two events is required for an understanding of the structural changes brought about by flexion. The two remaining events will be described subsequently.

THE NERVOUS SYSTEM AND MESODERMAL SOMITES

THE NEURAL PLATE

Early in the third week of gestation the ectodermal cells become taller in the interval between the primitive node and the oral plate. They constitute the slipper-shaped *neural plate* (Fig. 6-1). The broader, rostral, part—the *brain plate*—will form the brain, while the spinal cord will be derived from the remainder. The neural plate includes the neurenteric canal in its floor.

SEGMENTATION OF THE MESODERM

The mesoderm beside the notochord (or axis) is known as the *paraxial mesoderm.* It increases in thickness, and its cells aggregate to form a series of cell blocks, or *somites.* The first pair of somites appears at the junction of the brain and spinal cord primordia on the 20th day. Segmentation of the paraxial mesoderm continues during the following ten days, successive pairs of somites appearing behind the first.

The mesoderm beside the brain plate does not take part in segmentation. Lateral to the somites the mesoderm also remains unsegmented. The strip adjacent to the somites is called the *intermediate mesoderm* (Fig. 6-2). External to this is the *lateral plate mesoderm,* which contains the coelom. The lateral plate is subdivided into the *somatic mesoderm,* which lies

38

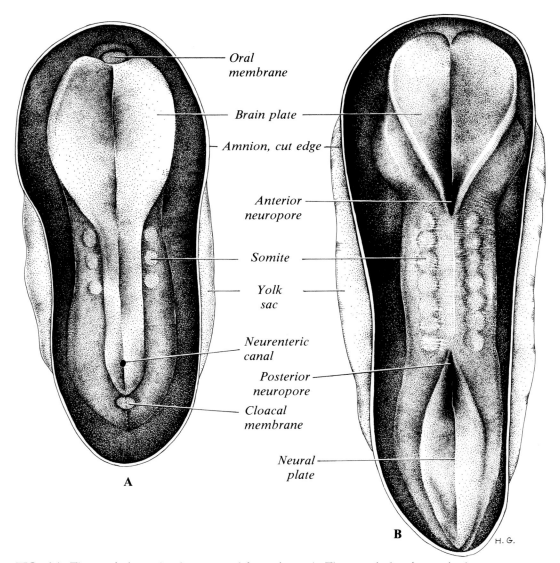

FIG. 6-1. The amniotic sac has been opened from above. **A.** The neural plate is seen in the floor of the sac, flanked by three pairs of somites visible through the skin ectoderm (cf Fig. 6-3). (Adapted from Ingalls NW; Contrib Embryol Carnegie Inst 11:61–90, 1920)
B. The neural folds have united at the middle of the embryo; seven pairs of somites are seen through the skin ectoderm. The neural plate is open at each end of the embryo. (Adapted from Payne F: Contrib Embryol Carnegie Inst 16:117–124, 1924)

FIG. 6-2. Formation of the neural tube.

against the amnion, and the *splanchnic mesoderm,* which lies against the yolk sac (Fig. 6-2B). The somatic mesoderm and the related amnion are together known as the *somatopleure.* The splanchnic mesoderm and related endoderm form the *splanchnopleure.*

THE NEURAL TUBE

As the paraxial mesoderm thickens progressively the neural plate overlying it becomes elevated on each side to form *neural folds* (Figs. 6-2 and 6-3). The thinner epithelium on the lateral aspect of each neural fold is the *skin ectoderm,* as distinct from the *neurectoderm* on the medial slope (Fig. 6-2B).

The segmenting mesoderm projects dorsally, raising the neural folds and thrusting them together in the median plane. The neurectoderm contributes to the folding process by actively altering the shape of its component cells. The neural folds meet to form the *neural tube.* Neurectoderm joins neurectoderm, and skin ectoderm joins skin ectoderm. The two ectodermal elements then separate from one another, so that the neural tube is ventral to the skin ectoderm. Fusion of the folds begins at the level of the earlier somites and progresses rapidly in rostral and caudal directions. The open ends of the neural tube (Fig. 6-1B) are the *anterior* and *posterior neuropores.*

THE NEURAL CREST

As the neural folds approach one another, the cells at the *crest* of the neurectoderm, *i.e.,* adjacent to its junction with skin ectoderm, escape from the folds and come to lie dorsolateral to the completed neural tube. Here they form the *neural crest* (Fig. 6-2C). Segmentation of the mesoderm induces the neural crest to break up into individual cell groups corresponding to the somites.

FIG. 6-3. Transverse section of an embryo in the early somite period. (Cambridge Collection) (x130)

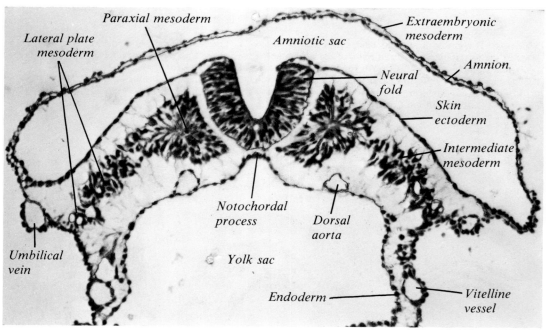

FORMATION OF THE HEAD AND TAIL FOLDS: THE PHENOMENON OF REVERSAL

Figure 5-5 shows that the septum transversum, which will contribute to the *diaphragm,* is as first rostral to the pericardial cavity, which will contain the *heart;* and this in turn is rostral to the oral membrane, the site of the *mouth.* It is clear that the attainment of the adult anatomic arrangement demands a reversal of the relative sequence of the septum, cavity, and membrane. The cloacal membrane (*cloaca,* a sewer) will cover the *anal* and *urinary* outlets, and the caudal mesoderm will form the *infraumbilical abdominal wall.* Here, too, the relative order anticipates a process of reversal.

The septum transversum is the relatively fixed part about which the *head fold* is formed. The caudal mesoderm is the corresponding fulcrum for the *tail fold.* In the sagittal section shown in Figure 6-4A it can be seen that folding of the embryo is already under way. The pericardial cavity is dorsal to the septum transversum, and the oral membrane is dorsal to the pericardium. The cloacal membrane is dorsal to the caudal mesoderm.

FIG. 6-4. Sagittal sections showing formation of the head and tail folds. **Arrows** in A and B indicate expansion of the amniotic sac.

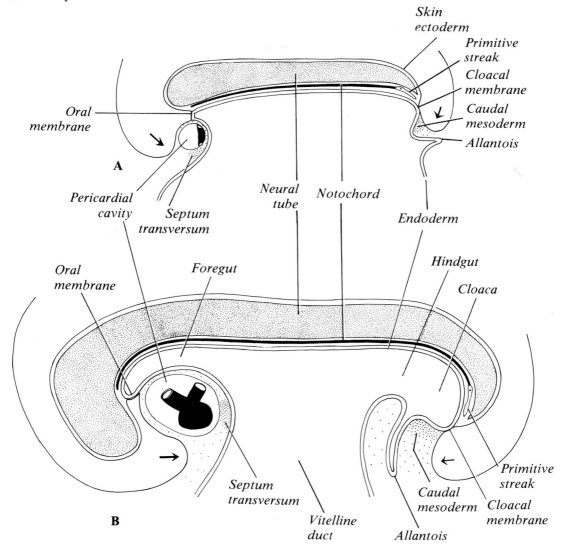

Figure 6-4B shows that folding has been completed. The septum transversum and caudal mesoderm, originally at opposite ends of the embryonic disk, are now close to one another, separated by the yolk sac and allantois. The developing brain is at the rostral extremity of the embryo, and the oral membrane lies between it and the pericardium. The septum transversum is immediately caudal to the pericardium, completing the "proper" (adult) anatomic sequence of parts. The caudal mesoderm now lies rostral to the cloacal membrane.

The relationship of body parts after folding is reviewed in Figure 6-5A. The position of the mouth is indicated, also that of the pericardium, the diaphragm (derived in part from septum transversum), and the lower abdominal wall (which receives a contribution from the caudal mesoderm).

Figure 6-6 is a photograph of the rostral part of a 25-day embryo. The oral membrane is well shown. The recess external to the membrane, lined by skin ectoderm, is the *stomodeum*. The caudal part of the section passes out of the plane of the foregut and neural tube to enter the plane of the somites.

THE LATERAL BODY FOLDS

Figure 6-7A shows a transverse section through the middle of the embryo, where the embryonic coelom is in communication with the extraembryonic coelom. Formation of the lateral body folds has already begun. The paraxial mesoderm has retained its position lateral to the neural tube and notochord, but the intermediate and lateral plate mesoderm have been deflected ventrally by the expanding amniotic sac. The embryonic coelom opens in a ventral direction on both sides. The yolk sac is being constricted by the splanchnic mesoderm.

Figure 6-7B shows the arrangement following completion of lateral folding, which could be visualized as being immediately rostral or caudal to the yolk sac constriction shown in Figure 6-4B. The paraxial mesoderm has remained *in situ*. The intermediate mesoderm bulges into the coelom. The two elements of the lateral plate have fused with their opposite numbers in the midline—splanchnic mesoderm has fused with splanchnic mesoderm to enclose the gut; and somatic mesoderm has met somatic mesoderm ventral to the embryonic coelom. The open parts of the embryonic coelom have joined to create the *peritoneal cavity*.

FIG. 6-5. Arrangement of parts in the eighth week of gestation: **A,** in sagittal section; **B,** in transverse section.

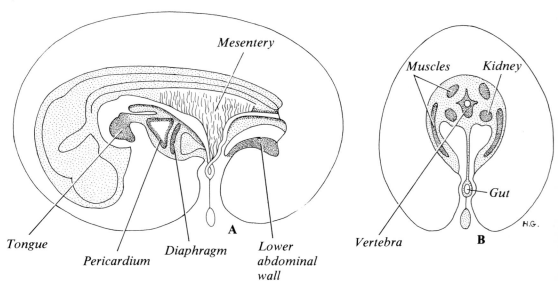

Mesentery

Muscles   Kidney

Gut

Tongue

Vertebra

Pericardium   Diaphragm   Lower abdominal wall

A   B

H.G.

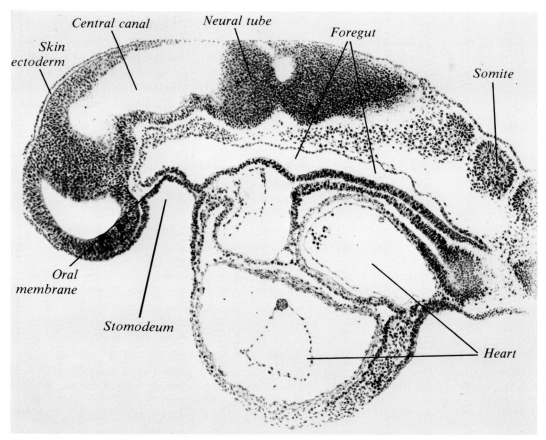

FIG. 6-6. Sagittal section of 25-day embryo. (Carnegie Collection) (x150)

FIG. 6-7. The lateral body folds: **A**, during folding; **B**, folding completed.

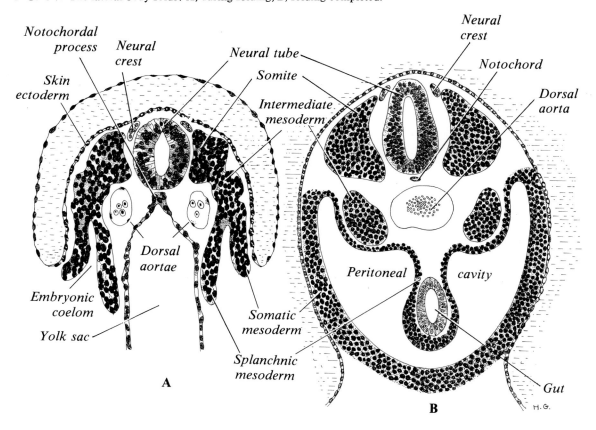

The fate of the relevant mesoderm is summarized in Figure 6-5B. The somites, in addition to forming the musculature of the trunk, build the vertebral column around the notochord and neural tube. The intermediate mesoderm forms the kidneys, suprarenal cortex, and gonads. The splanchnic mesoderm encloses the portion of the yolk sac that is retained within the embryo, giving it its muscle coat and mesentery. The somatic mesoderm contributes to the connective tissue of the wall of the trunk.

CHANGES IN THE AMNIOTIC SAC AND YOLK SAC

Folding of the embryo is associated with profound changes in the disposition of the amniotic sac and yolk sac. The amniotic sac expands progressively, so that when flexion is complete the entire embryo is invested by the skin ectoderm. This investment will later produce the epidermis of the skin. The embryo is enclosed henceforward in a protective bag of amniotic fluid (Fig. 6-8), which is secreted initially by the amniotic epithelium.

The yolk sac is constricted by the body folds, and comes to resemble an hourglass. The part of the yolk sac retained within the embryo elongates to form the *gut*. More specifically, it produces the lining epithelium of the alimentary tract. The part excluded from the embryo is the *yolk sac remnant* (Fig. 6-8); this shrinks during later pregnancy and can seldom be identified at birth. The connection between the gut and the yolk sac remnant is the *vitelline duct*. The *foregut* extends from the oral membrane to the cephalic limit of the vitellointestinal communication. *The embryonic foregut includes the future pharynx and esophagus.* It therefore differs from the foregut of adult anatomy, which reaches cranially only to the gastroesophageal junction. The *midgut* is the section opposite the vitelline duct. The *hindgut*

FIG. 6-8. Six-week embryo and membranes. (Carnegie Collection) (x3)

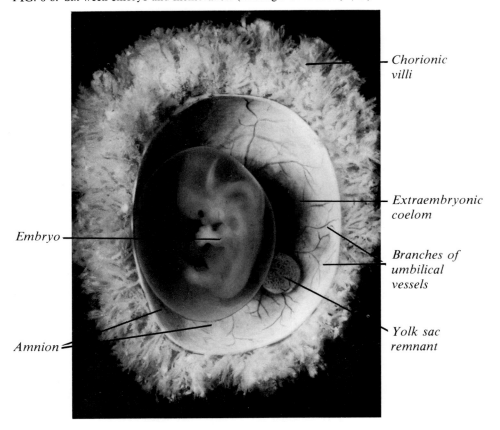

Chorionic villi

Extraembryonic coelom

Embryo

Branches of umbilical vessels

Yolk sac remnant

Amnion

continues caudally to reach the cloacal membrane. The part of the hingut that lies caudal to the allantoic diverticulum is the *cloaca* (Fig. 6-4B).

The significance of the term "septum transversum," used to designate the rostral mesoderm that lay cephalic to the pericardial cavity, is now apparent. It is a transverse partition separating the pericardial cavity from the endoderm at the junctional area between the foregut and the vitelline duct (Fig. 6-4B).

THE BRANCHIAL ARCHES

Beside the rostral end of the notochord, the paraxial mesoderm does not undergo segmentation. While the head fold increases, this mesoderm quickly fans out on the sides of the primitive brain and foregut. It invests the brain completely and infiltrates between the floor of the foregut and the pericardium. The cephalic part of the foregut thus enclosed is the *embryonic pharynx;* and here the mesoderm shows a succession of bilateral thickenings called the *branchial* (or *pharyngeal*) *arches.* The first pair to appear are the *mandibular arches,* in which the mandible will develop; they meet caudal to the stomodeum and abut against the pericardium. By the end of the third week the second and third pair of arches have appeared. They are parallel to the mandibular arches and they intervene between them and the developing heart. Later, two more pairs develop.

Neural crest cells adjacent to the hindbrain invade the branchial mesoderm and contribute to its cartilaginous derivatives. An artery develops within each arch, and motor nerves from the hindbrain grow in to supply the muscles that develop from the branchial mesoderm (Fig. 6-9).

Although the pharyngeal arches are purely mesodermal in composition, they are intimately related to the other germ layers. They raise external ridges visible through the covering ectoderm, and internal ridges on the sides and floor of the pharynx. The arches are homologous with the gill arches of fishes, but in mammals the interval between successive arches does not break down, *i.e.,* gill slits do not appear.

FIG. 6-9. Schematic section of a pair of branchial arches.

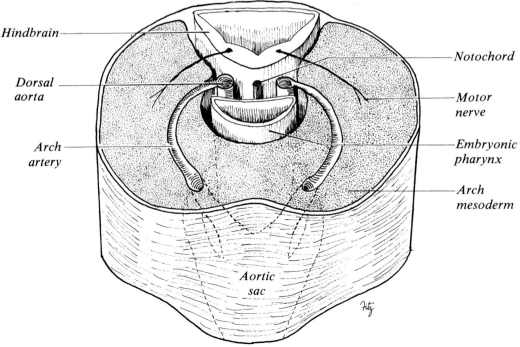

Hindbrain

Dorsal aorta

Arch artery

Notochord

Motor nerve

Embryonic pharynx

Arch mesoderm

Aortic sac

THE UMBILICAL CORD

The body stalk is initially broad and extends onto the dorsal aspect of the amniotic sac (Fig. 5-2). As the sac expands the body stalk and the contained allantois are displaced to the sac's ventral aspect (Fig. 6-10A). Both the stalk and the yolk sac become constricted (Fig. 6-10B). The appearance of a vascular system within the stalk completes the *umbilical cord,* which connects the ventral aspect of the embryo to the placenta. For a time the peritoneal cavity retains its communication with the extraembryonic coelom at the umbilicus. It will be seen later that the function of this communication is to permit coils of fetal intestine to be accommodated within the umbilical cord. The expanding amnion covers the umbilical cord, and the vitelline duct is incorporated into the cord (Fig. 6-10C). During this process the embryo rotates within the chorionic vesicle until its ventral surface faces the chorion frondosum.

CARDIOVASCULAR SYSTEM

VITELLINE VESSELS

In vertebrate ova rich in yolk an extensive plexus of *vitelline vessels* develops on the yolk sac. In higher mammals, whose ova are deficient in yolk, the placenta supersedes the yolk sac and the vitelline circulation, as such, is short-lived. The vitelline vessels, however, do not

FIG. 6-10. The chorionic vesicle: **A,** during the third week, **B,** during the fourth week; **C,** during the sixth week.

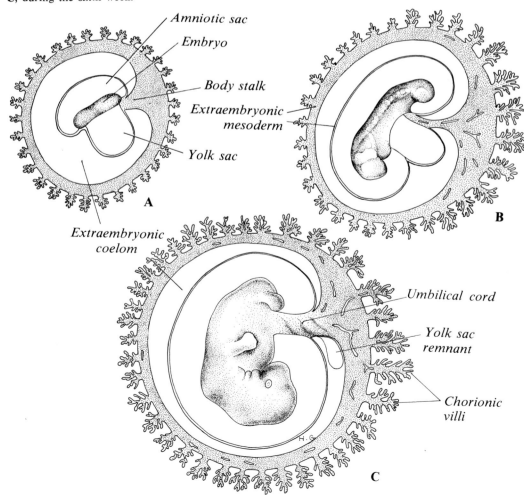

Amniotic sac

Embryo

Body stalk

Extraembryonic mesoderm

Yolk sac

A

B

Extraembryonic coelom

Umbilical cord

Yolk sac remnant

Chorionic villi

C

disappear; they are adapted to the arterial supply and venous drainage of the part of the yolk sac that is retained within the embryo, *i.e.,* the gut. Vitelline arteries supply the fore-, mid- and hindgut, and vitelline veins are the basis of the portal vein.

THE BLOOD ISLANDS

On the surface of the yolk sac, clusters of *hemangioblasts* differentiate from the extraembryonic mesoderm. They form two cell types—*hemocytoblasts,* occupying the center of each cluster, and peripheral *angioblasts,* which join one another to form flattened vascular endothelium and enclose the hemocytoblasts (Fig. 6-11). The hemocytoblasts constitute the *blood islands* of the embryo; they are the stem cells of the red and white corpuscles for the greater part of the embryonic period. The red cells produced in the blood islands retain their nuclei.

FIG. 6-11. Transverse section of a 23-day, 7-somite embryo. (Carnegie Collection) (x180)

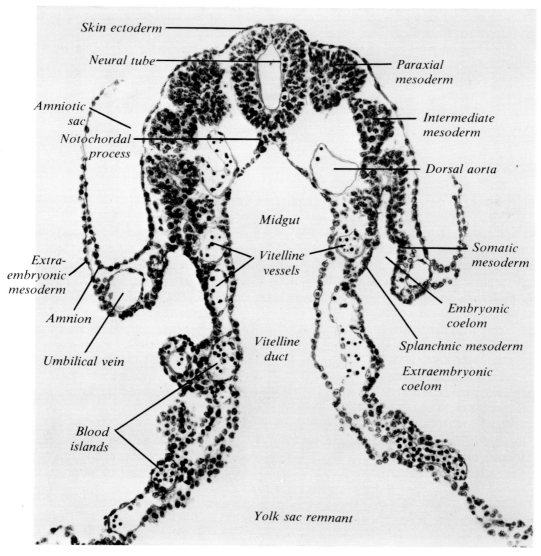

The angioblasts form an extensive capillary plexus on the yolk sac; the plexus buds dorsally to link up with the vitelline arteries and veins within the embryo, and they discharge the primitive blood cells into the embryonic circulation.

THE UMBILICAL VEINS

In the body stalk and chorion, angioblasts give rise to endothelial sacs similar to those on the yolk sac (but without blood islands). To gain the embryo the capillary buds extend ventral to the enlarging amniotic sac. They are thus conducted to the *somatic* embryonic mesoderm. As they reach towards the embryonic heart they run lateral to the vitelline vessels, being separated from them by the embryonic coelom (Fig. 6-11).

THE PRIMITIVE HEART

The entire heart has its origin in the splanchnic mesoderm that forms the floor of the pericardial cavity; this area is known as the *cardiogenic crescent.* Formation of the head fold rotates the entire rostral mesoderm through 180 degrees, and the cardiogenic crescent is transferred from the floor of the pericardial cavity to its roof.

The crescent gives rise to a pair of endothelial tubes. These unite to form the *primitive heart tube,* which projects into the pericardial cavity.

The caudal end of the heart tube abuts against the septum transversum. The vitelline and umbilical veins grow through the septum and enter it on each side. The cephalic end of the heart elongates to form the *truncus arteriosus,* whose distal end expands as the *aortic sac* (Fig. 6-9).

THE FETAL VESSELS

Dorsal Aortae

Capillary networks beside the notochord give rise to right and left *dorsal aortae.* The aortae are linked to the aortic sac by the first pair of aortic arterial arches (Fig. 6-12A), which pass through the mandibular mesoderm. Further pairs of aortic arches pass through the remaining branchial arches as these appear. From the point of union of the first arch artery with its dorsal aorta a narrow channel extends beneath the brain. This is the rudiment of the *internal carotid artery* (Fig. 6-12B).

From their dorsolateral aspects the aortae give off *intersegmental* arteries which pass between the somites to supply the differentiating mesoderm and neural tube. Numerous ventral, *vitelline* branches ramify on the surface of the yolk sac and establish connections with the vitelline plexus.

Two umbilical arteries extend from the dorsal aortae into the body stalk; they branch within the chorion and unite with vessels forming there.

Caudal to the aortic arches the dorsal aortae fuse to become a single, midline vessel, in the interval between notochord and gut (Figs. 6-7 and 6-12B). When the full complement of somites develops, fusion of the aortae is found to extend caudally from the fourth thoracic somite, and the umbilical arteries are attached to the aorta at the level of the fourth lumbar somite. Between these levels the aorta therefore forms the *descending thoracic* and the *abdominal aorta,* which span the interval between the fourth thoracic and the fourth lumbar vertebrae in the adult. The umbilical arteries tap the aortic blood when the circulation commences, and caudal to them the aorta fails to develop significantly. It persists here as the small *median sacral* artery.

The vitelline arteries come together in the midline; their number is reduced to three (Figs. 6-12B and 6-13).

The Cardinal Veins

The cardinal veins are the last major vessels to appear. They lie dorsolateral to the aortae, and they drain the nervous system and mesodermal somites. The veins of each side are *anterior* and *posterior,* and they unite to form the *common cardinal vein* (Fig. 6-12B) which joins the vitelline and umbilical veins at their point of entry into the heart.

THE EMBRYONIC CIRCULATION

The time when the human heart begins to beat is uncertain, but the information from comparative embryology places it at about 21 days following fertilization. The histogenesis of cardiac muscle need not be complete, for heart cells (chick) in tissue culture contract

FIG. 6-12. Embryonic vessels: **A**, initially paired; **B**, later partially fused. The intersegmental vessels are not shown. AS, aortic sac. (Adapted from Felix W: Morph Jarb 41:577, 1910)

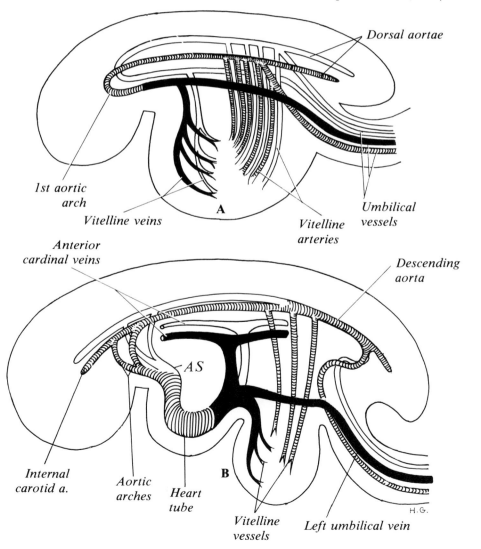

Dorsal aortae

1st aortic arch

Vitelline veins

A

Vitelline arteries

Umbilical vessels

Anterior cardinal veins

Descending aorta

AS

Internal carotid a.

Aortic arches

Heart tube

B

Vitelline vessels

Left umbilical vein

H.G.

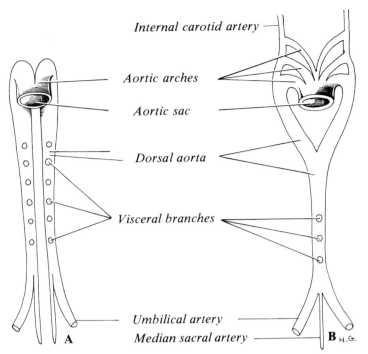

FIG. 6-13. Fusion of the paired dorsal aortae (**A**) to form the descending aorta (**B**) and the development of the internal carotid artery and the aortic arterial arches.

rhythmically before the characteristic cellular striations have appeared. From the heart tube, blood enters the aortic sac and flows through the branchial arches into the dorsal aortae. A small amount enters the internal carotid arteries to supply the brain, being returned in the anterior cardinal veins. The remainder is distributed to the three primary circulatory systems: 1) to the yolk sac (later, the gut) in the vitelline arteries, to be returned by the vitelline veins; 2) to the body wall and nervous system by the intersegmental arteries, to be returned by the cardinal veins; and 3) to the placenta by way of the umbilical arteries, returning in the corresponding veins.

THE SIGNIFICANCE OF PLEXUSES

The plexiform arrangement of the embryonic blood vessels is important in that it provides alternative channels for the circulating blood. The basic pattern of the vasculature is determined by genetic factors, but the maturation of individual vessels is influenced by blood flow. The most appropriate channel enlarges, and the more peripheral capillaries retract and disappear. Regional fluctuations arising from the position, growth rate, and the like, of organ rudiments determine the preferred channels. It is not surprising that variations in the manner of branching of the main vessels of the adult (*e.g.,* external carotid, subclavian, internal iliac, femoral), and in the course of the small vessels, are commonplace.

ANATOMIC REVIEW

Figure 6-14 represents a reconstruction of a 21-day embryo. The amniotic sac has been cut away to expose the embryo. The neural folds are shown in A and B. Beside the brain plate the *otic placode* (which will form the inner ear) is a thickening of the skin ectoderm. The embryonic coelom has appeared in the region of the heart tube; it has not yet extended into the lateral plate on either side. All around, the embryonic mesoderm blends with the investing extraembryonic mesoderm.

Parts C and D of Figure 6-14 show that the head fold of this embryo is well advanced, but the tail fold is only beginning. The pericardium is tucked under the foregut, and the heart tube is invaginating it. The artery of the first (mandibular) branchial arch has made its appearance; it links the heart tube to the corresponding dorsal aorta. The umbilical vessels are well developed in the body stalk; the arteries have joined the dorsal aortae but the veins have not yet budded into the embryo. Vitelline arteries are sprouting from the dorsal aortae to tap the blood islands on the wall of the yolk sac; the paired vitelline veins are meeting in the septum transversum to enter the heart tube.

The caudal mesoderm occupies its appropriate position dorsal to the allantois and caudal to the cloacal membrane. It blends with the extraembryonic mesoderm of the body stalk.

Figure 6-15 represents a reconstruction of a 24-day embryo. *An understanding of the anatomy of this embryo will provide a firm base for appreciation of regional embryonic development.* Folding is nearing completion, and the embryo is covered by the skin ectoderm. The paraxial mesoderm has formed 14 somites, and the mandibular arches have joined one another ventral to the pharynx (Fig. 6-15A). The embryonic coelom is open in the middle third of the embryo; it sends a *pelvic extension* caudally beside the hindgut; this will form the pelvic part of the peritoneal cavity (Fig. 6-15B).

The three components of the circulation (vitelline, umbilical, and cardinal) are present (Fig. 6-15C). The first and second branchial arch arteries pass to the dorsal aortae. Vitelline arteries ramify in profusion in the splanchnic mesoderm covering the yolk sac, the blood being returned in the right and left vitelline veins. The umbilical arteries enter the body stalk together with the allantois, carrying waste products to the placenta. The umbilical veins (carrying oxygenated blood) run cranially in the *somatic* mesoderm to reach the heart. The blood supply to the fetus itself is still poorly developed. Small intersegmental arteries (not shown) run between the somites to supply the neural tube; this blood is returned to the cardinal veins, which lie dorsal to the aortae and are not yet linked to the heart (Fig. 6-15C).

Foregut, midgut, and hindgut are easily identified. The vitelline duct is in wide communication with the yolk sac remnant, which has been cut away (Fig. 6-15D).

At the caudal extremity the primitive streak is adding to the caudal mesoderm by means of cells that migrate alongside the cloacal membrane. The caudal mesoderm in turn is extending rostrally past the allantois into the lower part of the abdominal wall (Fig. 6-15D).

Figure 6-16 shows the anatomy of the rostral part of the embryo depicted in Figure 6-15. The neural tube is open at the anterior neuropore and at its lips the neurectoderm is reflected into continuity with the skin ectoderm. The *optic recess* is a lateral outgrowth of the brain; it will form the optic nerve and retina.

The brain overhangs the developing heart, creating an ectoderm-lined recess, the stomodeum, which has the oral membrane in its roof. The pharynx reaches rostrally to the oral membrane. The endoderm in its floor shows three zones of proliferation: 1) the *thyroid diverticulum,* which is the precursor of the thyroid gland and grows into close relation to the aortic sac; 2) the *respiratory diverticulum,* which also buds ventrally from the pharynx, and will go on to form the lower part of the respiratory system; and 3) the *hepatic bud,* which will invade the septum transversum and form the liver and biliary tract.

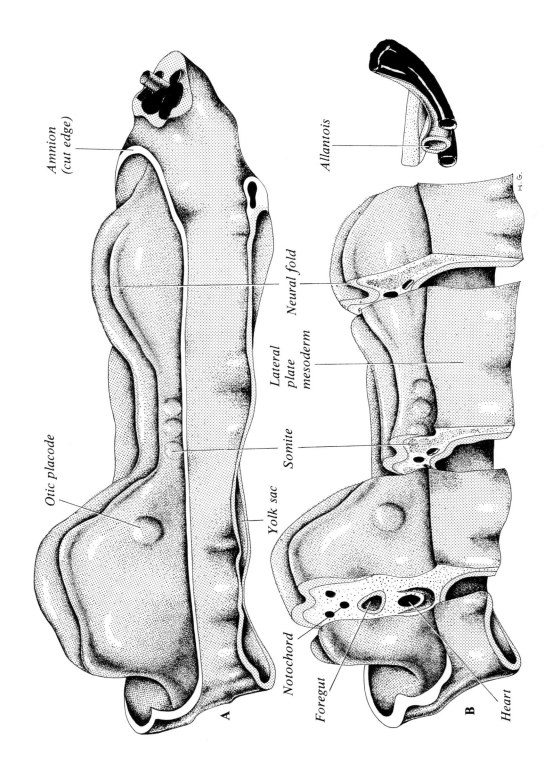

Amnion
(cut edge)

Allantois

Neural fold

Lateral
plate
mesoderm

Otic placode

Somite

Yolk sac

Notochord

Foregut

Heart

A

B

H. G.

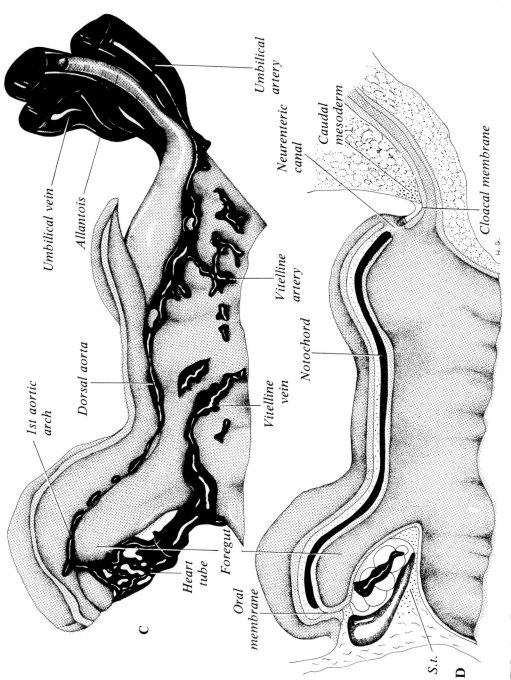

FIG. 6-14. Reconstructions of a three-somite embryo. **A**, Side view; **B**, stereosections; **C**, blood vessels, neural plate, gut; **D**, sagittal section. (Adapted from Ingalls NW: Contrib Embryol Carnegie Inst 11:61–90, 1920)

C labels: Umbilical artery, Umbilical vein, Allantois, Neurenteric canal, Vitelline artery, 1st aortic arch, Dorsal aorta, Vitelline vein, Heart tube, Foregut, Oral membrane, Notochord

D labels: Caudal mesoderm, Cloacal membrane, Notochord, S.t.

H.G.

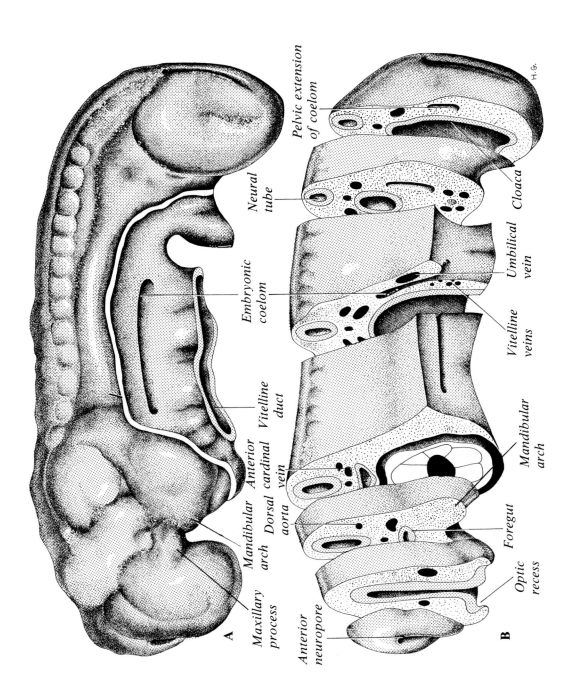

Pelvic extension
of coelom

Neural
tube

Cloaca

Embryonic
coelom

Umbilical
vein

Vitelline
veins

Vitelline
duct

Anterior
cardinal
vein

Mandibular
arch

Dorsal
aorta

Foregut

Maxillary
process

Optic
recess

Anterior
neuropore

A

B

H.G.

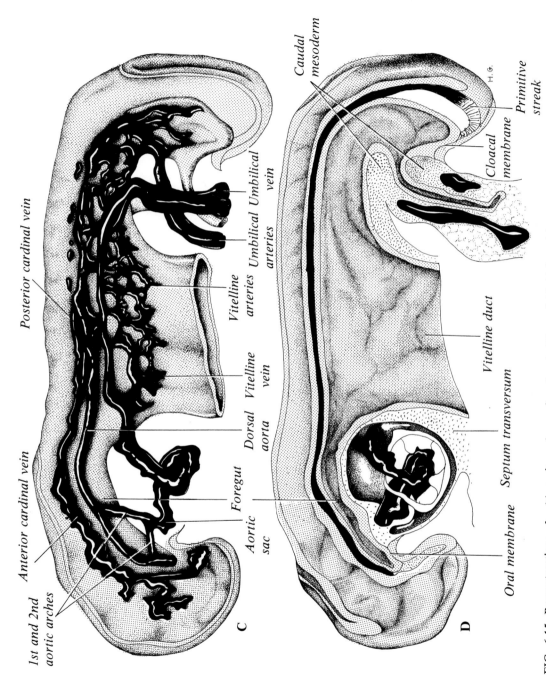

Posterior cardinal vein

Vitelline arteries Umbilical Umbilical vein arteries

Vitelline vein

Dorsal aorta

Foregut

Anterior cardinal vein

1st and 2nd aortic arches

Aortic sac

C

Caudal mesoderm

Cloacal membrane

Primitive streak

H. G.

Vitelline duct

Septum transversum

Oral membrane

D

FIG. 6-15. Reconstructions of a 14-somite embryo, viewed as in Figure 6-14. (Adapted from Heuser CH: Contrib Embryol Carnegie Inst 21:135–154,1930)

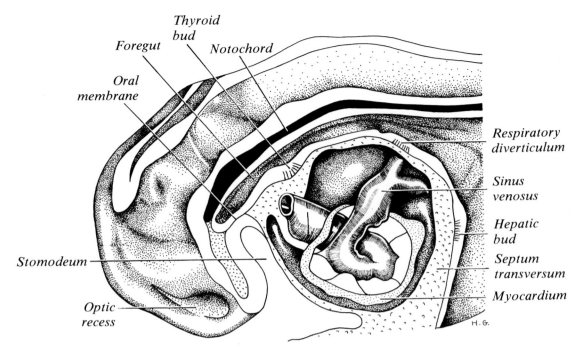

FIG. 6-16. The rostral part of the embryo shown in Figure 6-15.

SUGGESTED READING

Heuser CH: A human embryo with 14 pairs of somites. Contrib Embryol Carnegie Inst 21:135–154, 1930

Ingalls NW: A human embryo at the beginning of segmentation, with special reference to the vascular system. Contrib Embryol Carnegie Inst 11:61–90, 1920

Payne F: General description of a 7-somite human embryo. Contrib Embryol Carnegie Inst 16:117–124, 1924

Chapter 7

multiple pregnancy

The incidence of multiple pregnancy shows geographic and regional variation. At a rough estimate the incidence of twins is 1 in 85 pregnancies, triplets 1 in 85^2, and quadruplets 1 in 85^3.

TWINNING

Twins are of two kinds: *monovular, or identical;* and *binovular, or fraternal.*

Monovular twins develop from a single zygote, and therefore their genotypes are the same. Accordingly, they are of the same sex and resemble each other closely. Their blood groups are the same and their fingerprints are either similar or enantiomorphic *i.e.,* mirror images. However, the only absolute proof is the tolerance by one twin of a graft taken from the other. Monovular twinning is not hereditary.

Binovular twins result from the fertilization of two ova by separate spermatozoa. They may therefore be of the same or of opposite sex, and their genetic endowments are those of ordinary siblings. Fraternal twinning shows a hereditary tendency. It more commonly occurs in multipara, *i.e.,* in women who have already had one or more children, than in women who have not given birth previously. It may be described (not without offence) as a tendency to *litter*—multiple ovulation is the rule in lower animals.

TYPES OF MONOVULAR TWINS

There are three ways in which a single zygote may give rise to twins. Examination of the fetal membranes is usually sufficient to determine which mechanism is operative in a particular instance (Fig. 7-1).

Dichorial, Diamniotic Twins (Fig. 7-1A)

About 30% of twins are dichorial, diamniotic. In these the zygote divides in the normal manner, but at the two-cell stage the daughter cells separate and undergo independent development. Each cell is totipotent and gives rise to a complete individual. The two embryos implant and develop separately, behaving like fraternal twins.

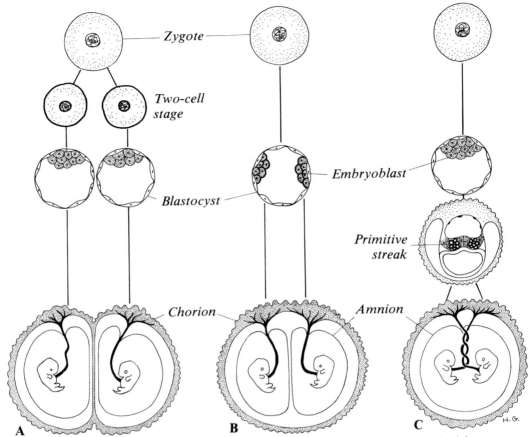

FIG. 7-1. Twinning: **A**, dichorial, diamniotic; **B**, monochorial, diamniotic; **C**, monochorial, monoamniotic.

Monochorial, Diamniotic Twins (Fig. 7-1B)

About 70% of twins are monochorial, diamniotic. In these twinning occurs within the blastocyst, the embryoblast being duplicated. Since the surrounding trophoblast forms the chorion both twins develop within one chorionic vesicle. Their placentas anastomose with one another to a variable extent. Rarely, the fetal vessels of one twin take a lion's share of the placental circulation. The other, progressively deprived of access to the maternal vascular bed, remains small and is grossly deformed; it usually becomes an *acardiac monster*.

Monochorial, Monoamniotic Twins (Fig. 7-1C)

About 1% of twins are monochorial, monoamniotic. In these two primitive streaks develop side by side. The single amniotic sac invests both embryos. The yolk sac is divided in two by the pinching-off process that normally accompanies lateral flexion of the embryo. The placental circulations anastomose. In most of this group the two umbilical cords become intertwined, posing a serious threat to both fetuses during parturition.

THREE OR MORE FETUSES

The mode of origin of three or more fetuses is the same as that of twins. They may be identical or fraternal; the former group results from the repeated division of a single zygote.

ABNORMALITIES

CONJOINT TWINS

Conjoint twins occur in about 1% of monozygotic twin pregnancies. They all belong to the monochorionic, monoamniotic group. The extent of conjunction is variable. One extreme is represented by infants in whom one or more organs—pituitary, tongue, or other structures —are duplicated; the other extreme, by twins joined only by a pedicle of skin. However, it is possible to define two great classes: class 1, those with incomplete duplication of the primitive streak and class 2, those with incomplete duplication of germ layers.

In class 1 the primitive streak is not rodlike but is λ- or Y-shaped. It is single for some of its length, and the vertebral column and nervous system (at least) are single at that level (Fig. 7-2). The result is a *duplex monster,* incapable of survival after birth.

In class 2 the primitive streaks are separate and the embryonic axes are clearly defined. However, the germ layers are not completely separate, one or more regions of the body being derived from the germ layers of both embryos. *Siamese twins* result (Fig. 7-3).

Because of advances in diagnostic and surgical techniques, Siamese twins can frequently be separated.

TERATOMAS

Teratomas are the most baffling of all tumors found in man. They are tissue masses foreign to the organ in which they arise. They are found in children; most of them are malignant.

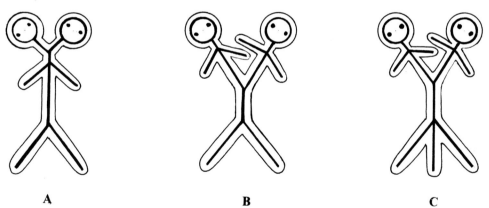

A B C

FIG. 7-2. Results of duplication of primitive streak: **A,** duplication of rostral end; **B,** duplication of rostral half; **C,** rostral and caudal duplication.

FIG. 7-3. Results of incomplete duplication of germ layers: **A,** rostrally; **B,** centrally; **C,** caudally.

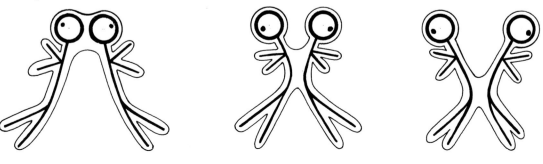

A B C

The neoplastic tissues comprise skin and its appendages, teeth, alimentary epithelium, and nervous tissue—all three germ layers usually contribute. About half the tumors occur in the testis or ovary; the rest tend to occupy the median plane in the sacral, cervical, or cranial regions.

Cytologic studies of *testicular* teratomas have demonstrated that nearly half are chromatin positive—a female character. This finding has led to the suggestion that teratomas may arise from the fusion of a pair of haploid (germ) cells within the testis or ovary of the developing embryo, the resultant diploid cell undergoing parthenogenetic development (*parthenos,* virgin). This hypothesis would account for chromatin-positive teratomas, assuming the union of two X-bearing cells. However, the sex chromatin may be found in some extragonadal teratomas in males.

The tendency for extragonadal teratomas to occur near the midline of the body indicates that they may have their origin in localized disorganization of germ layers in the region of the primitive streak and notochordal process, with later development of sequestered elements. This view would ally the condition to duplex monstrosity (class 1), the primitive streak or notochordal process undergoing grossly unequal division so that the second primordial embryo comes to be engulfed by the first (*fetus in fetu*).

SUGGESTED READING

Duhamel B, Haegel P, Pages R: Monstres doubles. In Morphogenese Pathologique. Paris, Masson, 1974, pp 223–273

Hendricks CH: Twinning in relation to birth weight, mortality, and congenital anomalies. Obstet Gynecol 27:47–53, 1966

Salerno LJ: Monoamniotic twinning. Obstet Gynecol 14:205–213, 1959

Stevens LC, Pierce GB: Teratomas: definitions and terminology. In Sherman MI, Salter D (eds): Teratomas and Differentiation. New York, Academic Press, 1975, pp 13–16

Taylor A: The status of the teratoma: studies in sex chromosome distribution. In The Early Conceptus, Normal and Abnormal. Baltimore, Williams & Wilkins, 1965, pp 78–80

Chapter 8

spinal cord and body wall

THE SPINAL CORD

As the neural folds come together the neurectodermal cells form a pseudostratified epithelium extending from inner to outer surfaces (limiting membranes) of the neural tube. The cell nuclei are dispersed evenly at first, but they quickly retire towards the central canal. In the inner, *ventricular zone* (or *ependymal zone*) the cells divide, and as they do so they become detached from the limiting membranes. However, some maintain their attachments to provide a scaffolding for the outward migration of daughter cells.

The daughter cells are of two kinds, nervous and neuroglial. Both complete their differentiation in the *intermediate* or *mantle zone* of the neural tube (Fig. 8-1A).

THE NERVE CELLS

The *neuroblasts,* or presumptive nerve cells, emit axonal processes. The first to do so are the motor neuroblasts of the future *ventral (anterior) horn* of gray matter. Their axons emerge from the neural tube (as the anterior nerve root) and make prompt contact with the nearest myotome. Following contact, dendrites develop and the nerve cells assume multipolar form. The expanding mass of motor neurons creates a bulge in the ventrolateral wall of the central canal (Fig. 8-1B). The resulting groove just dorsal to it is the *sulcus limitans*. The intermediate zone ventral to the sulcus is called the *basal plate,* and the zone dorsal to it is the *alar plate*. The neurons in the basal plate are predominantly *efferent,* or motor, and those in the alar plate are predominantly *afferent,* or sensory.

The alar plate gives rise to the *dorsal (posterior) horn* of gray matter (Fig. 8-1C). In the thoracic and upper lumbar regions an additional horn, the *lateral horn,* develops. The ventral part of the lateral horn, occupying the basal plate, is efferent; its axons emerge in the anterior nerve root and pass to the sympathetic ganglia. Its dorsal part is afferent and lies in the alar plate. Accordingly, it is possible to speak of four longitudinal cell columns in the gray matter on each side of the cord (Fig. 8-2). The *somatic efferent* column contains the motor cells whose axons supply the skeletal muscle derived from the mesodermal somites. The *visceral efferent* column contains the preganglionic motor neurons of the sympathetic nervous system. The *visceral afferent* column receives impulses from the thoracoabdominal viscera by way of the dorsal nerve roots. The *somatic afferent* column is played upon by impulses from the derivatives of the dermomyotomes.

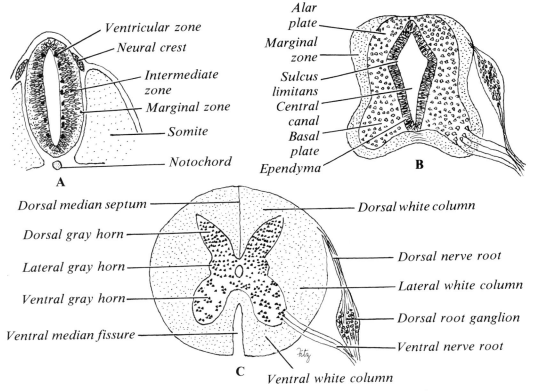

FIG. 8-1. Development of the spinal cord: **A**, fourth week; **B**, seventh week; **C**, newborn.

The enlarging anterior horns project ventrally, creating the *ventral median fissure.* The posterior horns approach each other, obliterating the posterior half of the central canal and forming the *dorsal median septum* (Fig. 8-1C).

SEGMENTS OF THE SPINAL CORD

The neural tube displays transient bulges, called *neuromeres,* between successive somites. Neuromeres are also found in the brain stem. Mitotic activity within the neuromeres is relatively high.

The *differentiated* central nervous system shows no evidence of segmentation. In clinical parlance, the term "spinal cord segment" refers to the nerve cell groups connected to the corresponding spinal nerve. There is no interruption of the cell columns between one "segment" and the next. The nerve roots emerge from the cord in a continuous series; they are secondarily collected into bundles which innervate the individual mesodermal somites.

NEUROGLIA

The parent cells are called *gliablasts.* They give rise to *astroblasts* and *oligodendroblasts.* The former become protoplasmic or fibrillar *astrocytes,* the latter become *oligodendrocytes.* The third neuroglial element, the *microglia,* is of mesodermal origin; these cells accompany the blood vessels that invade the nervous system.

As cytodifferentiation nears completion the ventricular zone is greatly reduced. The cells that remain there develop cilia and form the *ependyma* surrounding the central canal.

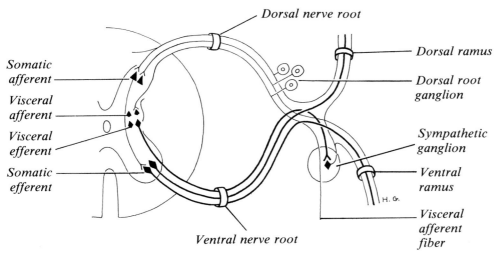

FIG. 8-2. Cell columns of the spinal cord and their connections.

CONNECTIONS OF SPINAL NEURONS

The outer, *marginal zone* of the neural tube is the basis of the white matter of the central nervous sytsem. During the second month it is increasingly invaded by central processes of the dorsal root ganglion cells. In addition to making local connections in the gray matter, the central processes send long ascending fibers to the hindbrain; these form the *dorsal white columns*. In the third month, intersegmental, bulbospinal, spinothalamic, and spinocerebellar neurons connect the various levels of the spinal cord with the brain, making up the *lateral* and *ventral white columns*. The pyramidal tracts—the newest fiber system phylogenetically—are the last to develop, in the fifth month. As the nerve tracts appear, neuroglial cells become dispersed among them.

Myelination commences in the fourth month and follows the order of appearance of the tracts. In the pyramidal tract it is not completed until 18 months after birth. Simple reflexes can be elicited before myelination has begun. During the third month of gestation the human fetus has been shown to respond to stroking of the face by an upward movement of the arm.

FATE OF THE NEURAL CREST

The neural crest is pluripotent, *i.e.,* it gives rise to tissues of more than one kind, and many of its cells have a remarkable migratory capacity. It gives rise to the following structures:

1. The *dorsal root ganglia* of the spinal nerves, and (in part) of their cranial nerve homologues. The ganglionic nerve cells are initially bipolar; their central processes enter the spinal cord while their peripheral processes mingle with those emerging from the anterior gray horn, to complete the spinal nerves. The ganglionic cells become unipolar by the union of their processes at one side of each cell.
2. Possibly, the *pia and arachnoid mater*. Alternatively, the pia-arachnoid may be delaminated from the surface of the neural tube.
3. The sheath cells of peripheral nerves—the *satellite cells* of ganglia and the *neurolemma* (Schwann sheath) of nerve fibers. At first each neurolemmal cell enfolds a large number of axis cylinders, but as the cells multiply they penetrate the nerve bundles. The coarser

fibers ultimately become the property of individual neurolemmal cells disposed in series along them. These fibers undergo myelinization by a remarkable "jelly-roll" movement of the cell membranes; the myelin sheaths are composed of layer upon layer of membrane lipoprotein. The finest fibers do not become myelinated; they are retained in groups by individual neurolemmal cells.

4. *Ganglia of the autonomic nervous system.* Neuroblasts migrate from the thoracic and upper lumbar levels of the neural crest to the sides and front of the vertebral column, to form the nerve cells of the sympathetic chain and of the intermediate abdominal ganglia (coeliac, mesenteric, renal). Axons grow out from them to innervate the cardiovascular, respiratory, intestinal, and genitourinary systems. The axons remain unmyelinated and constitute the *postganglionic* element of the sympathetic nervous system. *Preganglionic* fibers travel to the ganglia from the visceral efferent cell column; these become myelinated.

Parasympathetic ganglia arise by the migration of neurons to a position close to or within the organs they supply. Whether the neural crest contributes to them or whether they arise entirely by cell migration from the visceral efferent cell column is uncertain.

5. *Chromaffin tissue.* Some sympathetic neuroblasts fail to produce processes. The bulk of these cells become segregated as the *chromaffin cells* of the medulla of the suprarenal gland. Others form the *abdominal paraganglia,* which atrophy shortly after birth.

FIG. 8-3. Transverse section through the caudal part of an embryo in the fifth week. (Carnegie Collection) (x180)

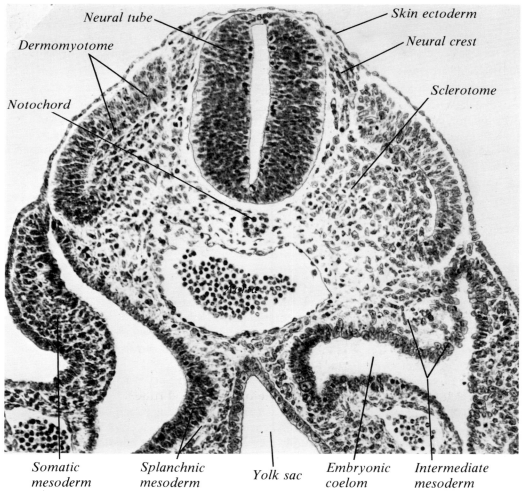

Neural tube — Skin ectoderm

Dermomyotome — Neural crest

Sclerotome

Notochord

Somatic mesoderm   Splanchnic mesoderm   Yolk sac   Embryonic coelom   Intermediate mesoderm

6. The *melanoblasts* of pigment-bearing skin and mucous membranes. These cells stream along sensory nerves to reach their target areas during the third month. The production and liberation of melanin are slow; Negro children are quite pale-skinned at birth, becoming darker during the first six postnatal weeks.
7. *Cartilage* within the branchial arches. The cells contributing to branchial arch cartilage are called *mesectodermal*.

THE BODY WALL

The ventromedial cells of the mesodermal somites lose their epithelioid character and become motile. This motile mesenchyme is the *sclerotome*. The remaining, dorsolateral half of the somite is the *dermomyotome* (Fig. 8-3).

THE SCLEROTOMES

The sclerotomes migrate medially, and opposite pairs meet around the notochord. The primordial vertebrae so formed are segmental in position, *i.e.,* they are at the same level as the dermomyotomes, and the intersegmental arteries run between them. By a remarkable transformation the sclerotomes combine to form the definitive vertebrae, which are bisegmental.

The sequence of events is followed in Figure 8-4: **A.** The cells in the caudal halves of the sclerotomes become close-packed. **B.** The primordial vertebrae fuse to provide a continuous mesenchymal pillar surrounding the notochord. **C.** The close-packed cells condense further and migrate rostrally until they lie opposite the center of the myotome above. **D.** These cells lay down alternating concentric and vertical layers of collagen to form the *intervertebral disks*. The notochord expands within each disk to form the gelatinous *nucleus*

FIG. 8-4. Stages in development of vertebrae and intervertebral disks. Three myotomes are represented at each margin.

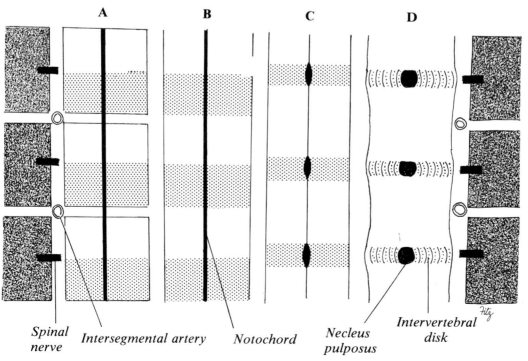

Spinal nerve   Intersegmental artery   Notochord   Necleus pulposus   Intervertebral disk

pulposus. The interval between successive disks is occupied by the *centrum* of the future vertebra. The centrum is bisegmental, its waist lying opposite the space between two successive myotomes. The intersegmental artery runs around the waist, and the spinal nerve is at the level of the disk.

From each centrum a *neural arch* grows back to enclose the spinal cord. The neural arch in turn gives off 1) the *spine,* where the two halves of the neural arch meet; 2) *transverse processes,* projecting between adjacent myotomes; and 3) *costal processes,* which grow ventrally in the somatic mesoderm (Fig. 8-5). The dura mater is delaminated from the inner surface of the neural arch mesenchyme.

In the sixth week, centers of chondrification appear in the centrum, neural arch, and costal processes. Chondrification spreads until a *cartilaginous vertebral column* has been completed. In the thoracic region, mesenchyme persists at the costovertebral junctions for the formation of synovial joints (Fig. 8-6).

In the eighth week, ossification centers appear at the original sites of chondrification (Fig. 8-7). At birth the vertebral centra, neural arches, and ribs are incompletely ossified. Each pair of *neurocentral synchondroses* lies within the main mass, or *body,* of the vertebra, and the ribs articulate only with neural arch elements (Fig. 8-8). At puberty the ossification of the vertebral spines and transverse processes, and of the heads and tubercles of the ribs, is completed from epiphyseal centers.

Only in the thorax do the costal processes and neural arches part company. In the cervical and lumbar regions the costal processes form the bulk of the "transverse processes" of adult anatomy. Their contribution to the sacrum is shown in Figure 8-9.

FIG. 8-5. Coronal section of vertebral region at five weeks. (Cambridge Collection) (x30)

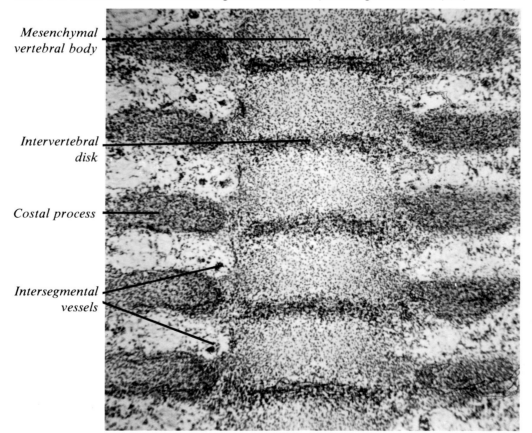

Mesenchymal vertebral body

Intervertebral disk

Costal process

Intersegmental vessels

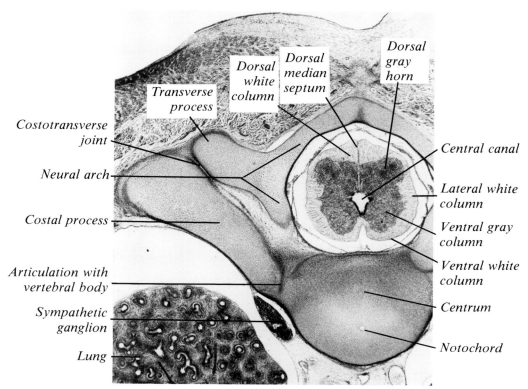

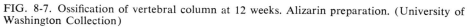

FIG. 8-6. The vertebral region in a 10-week fetus. (Carnegie Collection) (x30)

FIG. 8-7. Ossification of vertebral column at 12 weeks. Alizarin preparation. (University of Washington Collection)

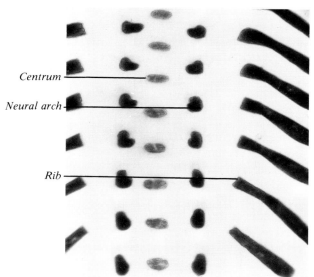

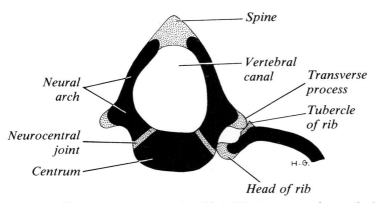

FIG. 8-8. Thoracic vertebra and rib at birth. **Black** represents bone; **stipple,** cartilage.

FIG. 8-9. The costal elements (black) at successive vertebral levels. The vertebral centra are in light stipple; the neural arches in darker stipple.

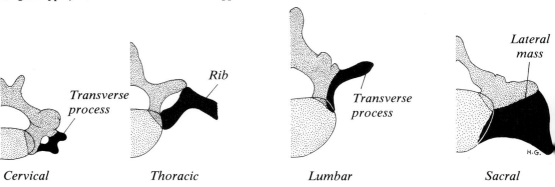

The centrum of the *atlas* fuses with that of the *axis* to form the *odontoid process.* The *hypochordal bow,* a transverse condensation of mesenchyme that contributes to the ligaments of the costovertebral joints elsewhere in the vertebral column, enlarges in the atlas to form its *anterior arch.*

ASCENT OF THE SPINAL CORD

Until the third month the spinal cord and meninges fill the vertebral canal and the nerve roots run directly to the intervertebral foramina. The later growth of the vertebral column outstrips that of the spinal cord. The upper end of the cord being fixed by its attachment to the brain, the lower part progressively ascends the vertebral canal. At the time of birth the tapered tip (*conus medullaris*) is at the level of the third lumbar vertebra. The dura and arachnoid mater continue to extend to the middle of the sacral canal; they enclose a pool of cerebrospinal fluid which can be sampled for diagnostic purposes without fear of injury to the spinal cord (Fig. 8-10). The anterior and posterior nerve roots now run obliquely to their points of union at the intervertebral foramina. The sacral and lower lumbar roots form the *cauda equina,* which floats in the subarachnoid space below the spinal cord.

The embryonic spinal cord is attached to the coccyx by neuroglia. This attachment is retained to form the *filum terminale* as the cord ascends (Fig. 8-10).

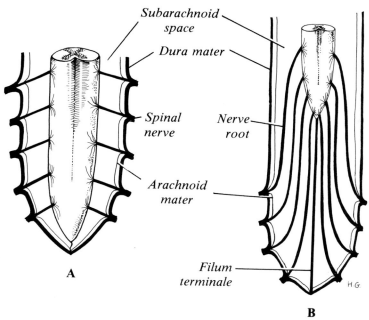

FIG. 8-10. Ascent of spinal cord: **A**, before; **B**, after.

THE DERMOMYOTOMES

When the sclerotome leaves its parent somite, the dermomyotome remaining elongates dorsoventrally and splits into *dermatome* and *myotome* (Chart 8-1). The dermatome applies

CHART 8-1. SUBDIVISIONS OF THE EMBRYONIC MESODERM IN THE TRUNK REGION

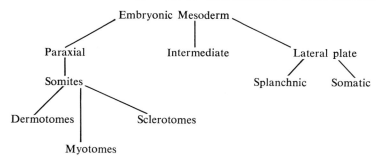

itself to the adjacent ectoderm and moves ventrally together with it during lateral flexion of the embryo. The dermatomes form the dermis of the skin; they retain their segmental innervation from the sensory (dorsal nerve root) component of the spinal nerves.

The myotome divides into a dorsal portion, or *epimere,* and a ventral *hypomere.* The spinal nerve splits into a *dorsal ramus* that innervates the muscles derived from the epimere, and a *ventral ramus* that supplies those derived from the hypomere. The epimeres join to form the primordium of the *erector spinae* muscle mass. The hypomeres migrate into the lateral plate mesoderm and give rise to the musculature of the neck and trunk.

The body wall muscles differentiate from the hypomere in three primary layers, the ventral ramus of the spinal nerve lying between the middle and innermost layers. Their segmental nature is well preserved in the intercostal muscles and is indicated elsewhere by their serial innervation. The external layer forms the *scalenus posterior* in the neck, the *external intercostals* in the thorax, and the *external oblique* in the abdomen. The middle layer forms the *scalenus medius, internal intercostals,* and *internal oblique.* The innermost layer, in addition to forming the *scalenus anterior, innermost intercostal* layer, and *transversus abdominis,* gives rise to the deepest muscles of the neck and trunk (*longus capitis, longus cervicis, quadratus lumborum, levator ani*).

ANTERIOR BODY WALL

In the thoracic region the ventral ends of the upper six costal processes become connected on each side of the midline by condensations of somatic mesoderm. The connections undergo chondrification to form two vertical *sternal bars,* which fuse from above downwards to form the cartilaginous *sternum* (Fig. 8-11). Commonly, fusion of the lower end is incomplete and the xiphoid process remains bifid or perforated. The sternum is later ossified from single or paired centers in the manubrium and body.

Near the midline the somatic mesoderm may contribute pre-muscle cells to the advancing myotomes, assisting them in forming the *rectus* musculature—the rectus abdominis, the infrahyoid "strap" muscles, and (when present) the ribbonlike *sternalis.*

The infraumbilical abdominal wall differs from the body wall elsewhere in requiring a direct contribution from the caudal mesoderm. With the completion of the tail fold the caudal mesoderm occupies the ventral aspect of the embryo rostral to the cloacal membrane (Fig. 6-15). Here it contributes to the external genitalia. It also spreads rostrally to form the somatic mesoderm of the lower abdominal wall, pushing the allantois and umbilical vessels ahead of it. The myotomes advance into the space thus created.

DEVELOPMENT OF THE UMBILICUS

Figure 8-12A presents a ventral view of the embryo shown in Figure 6-15. The amnion is attached to the skin ectoderm, which is advancing together with the underlying somatic mesoderm. The vitelline duct is invested with splanchnic mesoderm containing the vitelline vessels. On each side the embryonic coelom opens ventrally into the extraembryonic coelem. Caudally, the umbilical vessels and allantois occupy the umbilical cord. From the cord the umbilical veins travel in the somatic mesoderm to reach the heart.

Figure 8-12B shows the arrangement at the end of the fourth week. The somatopleure has advanced to make contact with the vitelline duct and body stalk; and between these two the embryonic coelom of the two sides communicates across the midline.

FIG. 8-11. Development of ribs and sternum: **A**, sixth week; **B**, seventh week; **C**, ninth week. (Adapted from Bardeen CR: In Keibel F, Mall FP [eds]: Manual of Human Embryology. Philadelphia, JP Lippincott, 1910, p 342)

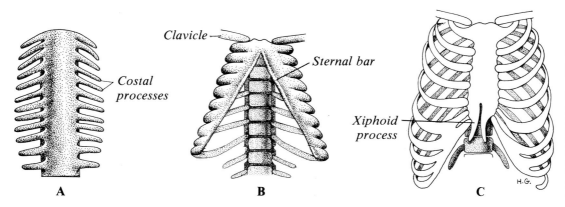

A   B   C

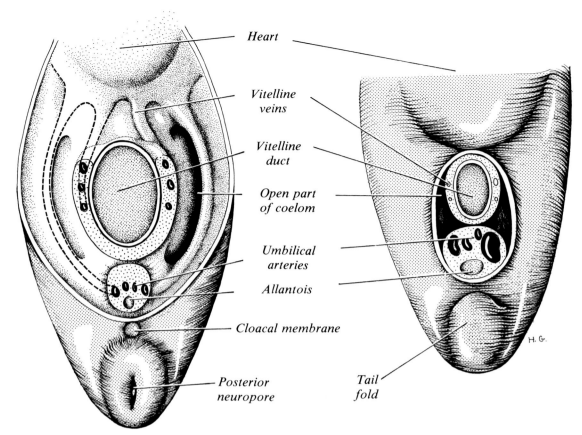

Heart

Vitelline veins

Vitelline duct

Open part of coelom

Umbilical arteries

Allantois

Cloacal membrane

Posterior neuropore

Tail fold

H. G.

FIG. 8-12. Ventral views of the embryo: **A**, at 24 days; **B**, at 28 days. The umbilical veins are not labeled.

The vitelline duct and yolk sac remnant atrophy during the embryonic period and the somatopleure advances to surround the umbilical cord. The area surrounded by the somatopleure during the fetal period is the *umbilicus*. It contains the umbilical cord together with a pouchlike extension of the embryonic coelom. Into this pouch, coils of intestine are extruded for a period of several weeks, creating the remarkable "physiological hernia of the midgut" (Ch. 11). During the first postnatal week the umbilicus is sealed off by the migration of skin ectoderm over the stump of the umbilical cord.

FATE OF THE INTERSEGMENTAL ARTERIES

In the neck the intersegmental arteries atrophy, their territory being taken over by the longitudinal *vertebral artery*. In the thorax the long costal processes and their attendant myotomes attract side branches that enlarge to become the *intercostal arteries*. In the lumbar region they persist unchanged, as the *lumbar arteries*. Below this level their points of origin are taken over by the internal iliac artery, from which they emerge as its *lateral sacral* branches.

THE SKIN AND ITS APPENDAGES

The epithelial structures of the skin are derived from the ectoderm. The dermis develops as a thickening of the dermatomes, which migrate through the somatic mesoderm and take up their position beneath the ectoderm.

During the second month the cuboidal skin ectoderm becomes two-layered. The superficial, *periderm* layer is shed as the epidermis differentiates; the deep, *germinal* layer forms the epithelial structures of the skin.

71

In the third month the germinal layer produces the stratified epithelium characteristic of mature epidermis. From the basal layer, epithelial pegs extend into the thickening dermis, and induce the formation of vascular mesodermal *dermal papillae*. Each peg forms a *hair bulb* around its papilla. A core of cells ascends from the bulb, differentiating into the keratinous hair shaft and its investing *inner root sheath* epithelium. The epidermal cells overlying each young hair die to create a canal for the hair. The first, fine hair coat is called *lanugo*. It is shed shortly before or after birth and coarser, *vellus hair* succeeds it. The vellus is largely derived from a second set of hair follicles.

In the fifth month of gestation the *sebaceous glands* bud into the dermis from the outer root sheath. They are holocrine in nature, entire cells being shed into the hair canal. The sebaceous secretion mixes with the discarded periderm to form the *vernix caseosa* ("cheesy varnish"), which is thought to preserve the fetus from the macerating effect of its fluid environment. The *sweat glands* develop at the same time as the sebaceous glands.

THE BREAST

In the sixth week a thickening of skin ectoderm, the *mammary ridge* or *milk line,* extends from axilla to groin on each side. In man, a single breast develops from its cranial part and the remainder disappears. In some mammals (*e.g.,* cat, dog, pig), breasts develop at intervals along the line, and in others (cow, sheep, deer) they develop only from the caudal third.

The human breast develops by an inward sprouting of 15–25 cords that slowly hollow out to become *lactiferous ducts*. The original thickening becomes depressed below the surface until, in the neonatal period, it grows to form the nipple.

In girls, glandular acini develop from the duct system at the time of pubertal breast enlargement. Some acini may be already formed at birth, however, and lactogenic hormone from the mother may cross the placenta and cause acini to secrete so-called "witch's milk" for a few days after the infant's birth.

ABNORMALITIES

VERTEBRAL ANOMALIES

Minor variation in the number of vertebrae is not uncommon. Such variation generally takes the form of *sacralization* of the fifth lumbar vertebra (giving rise to a sacrum with six vertebrae), or of *lumbarization* of the first sacral vertebra.

SPINA BIFIDA

The term "spina bifida" owes its origin to a failure of the neural arches to meet behind the spinal cord, the "bifid spine" being composed of the separated pairs of vertebral laminae. The condition usually occurs in the lumbosacral region. In its simplest form the defect is evident only on radiologic examination. This is *spina bifida occulta,* a frequent anomaly (1% of the population), which rarely causes symptoms.

Spina bifida cystica is a common malformation, with a prevalence of 1–4 per 1000 live births. One-quarter show anencephaly (see "Abnormalities" in Ch. 12) in addition. About 10% of cases are meningocoeles (Fig. 8-13A), in which the meninges protrude through a gap in the neural arches, usually in the lumbar region, and present as a cyst under the intact skin. The nervous system is usually normal. The remaining 90% are either *myelomeningocoeles* or *myelocoeles*. In a myelomeningocoele (Fig. 8-13B) the spinal cord, or cauda equina, floats within the cyst; neurologic deficits in the lower limb and bladder are common (Fig. 8-14). In a myelocoele (also known as *myeloschisis*) the neural tube fails to close in the lumbar region (Fig. 8-13C). Cerebrospinal fluid oozes over an open trough of neural tissue. The pelvic organs and lower limbs are paralysed and death ultimately follows infection of the nervous or urinary system.

Myelocoeles may show overgrowth of nervous tissue in the affected area, and this could possibly have prevented normal closure of the neural tube. However, the neural overgrowth could conceivably be a *result* of failure to close, rather than being the cause. A further possibility is a "blow-out" of the neural tube following normal closure. Such a rupture could be produced by a rise in pressure within the central canal should the escape routes (the foramina in the roof of the fourth ventricle) fail to appear at the normal time.

CERVICAL RIB

One or more additional ribs may result from elongation of cervical or lumbar costal processes. A *cervical rib,* attached to the seventh vertebra, may produce symptoms in adult life. It elevates and stretches the lower trunk of the brachial plexus, producing paralysis of the intrinsic muscles of the hand (which receive their nerve supply from the first thoracic segment of the spinal cord), vasomotor disturbance from interference with the sympathetic outflow to the limb, and loss of cutaneous sensation.

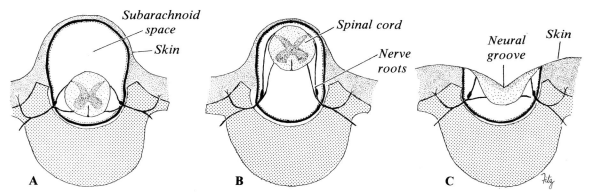

FIG. 8-13. Spina bifida cystica: **A**, meningocoele; **B**, myelomeningocoele; **C**, myelocoele.

FIG. 8-14. Myelomeningocoele. The lower limbs and bladder were paralysed. (Photograph kindly supplied by Dr F. W. L. Kerr.)

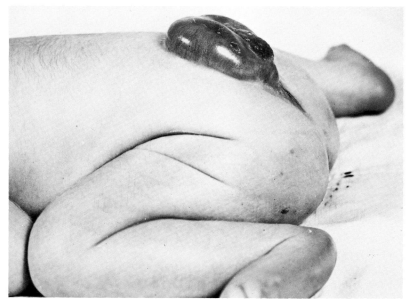

ABNORMAL DIFFERENTIATION OF THE NEURAL CREST

A normal complement of parasympathetic ganglia may fail to develop in the wall of the alimentary tract. In *Hirschsprung's disease* (*megacolon*) the distal large intestine displays an *aganglionic segment,* which fails to propagate peristaltic waves. The condition usually manifests itself by constipation and abdominal distension in infancy. Very surprisingly the innervation of the bladder is usually normal. In *congenital hypertrophic pyloric stenosis* the pyloric sphincter is greatly thickened, interfering with normal stomach emptying. The number of ganglion cells in the pyloric region is greatly reduced, but since the disease is cured by a simple incision of the sphincter, the changes in the intramural ganglia may not be primary.

Albinism is a congenital, hereditary condition characterized by absence of normal pigmentation from the skin and mucous membranes. The failure is not one of migration of melanoblasts, however, but of melanogenesis—deficiency of the enzyme *tyrosinase* interferes with the transformation of tyrosine to melanin.

GROWTH FAILURE IN THE SOMATOPLEURE

Exomphalos results from total failure of circumferential growth. The anterior abdominal wall is absent, and the peritoneal cavity and viscera are exposed.

If the primitive streak contribution to the infraumbilical abdominal wall is lacking, ectoderm and endoderm adhere, blocking the ventral advance of the regional myotomes and dermatomes. The area of adhesion breaks down, throwing the anterior part of the embryonic gut—which in this region forms the bladder—into open communication with the amniotic sac, creating so-called *exstrophy,* or *ectopia,* of the bladder.

In *congenital umbilical hernia* a coelomic loculus protrudes as a visible swelling. Minor degrees of umibilical hernia are commonplace; in these the somatopleure will complete its growth if the loculus is reduced by sustained pressure.

BREAST ANOMALIES

Absence of the nipples (and therefore of the breasts) is called *athelia. Polythelia* denotes the existence of supernumerary nipples; they may lie anywhere between axilla and groin, and rudimentary breasts may develop from them (polymastia*).

* *Mazon,* breast. The Amazons were women of the Tipuyas tribe who had the right breast cut off, the better to ply their bows and arrows.

SUGGESTED READING

Ambrose SS, O'Brien DP: Surgical embryology of the exstrophy-epispadias complex. Surg Clin North Am 54:1379–1390, 1974

Gardner WJ: Embryologic origin of spinal malformations. Acta Radiol [Diagn] (Stockh) 5:1013–1023, 1966

Jacobson M: Histogenesis and morphogenesis of the nervous system. In Jacobson M (ed): Developmental Neurobiology. New York, Holt, Rinehart & Winston, 1970, pp 1–64

Weston JA: The migration and differentiation of neural crest cells. In Abercrombie M, Brachet J, King TJ (eds): Advances in Morphogenesis, Vol 8. New York, Academic Press, 1970, pp 51–108

Wyburn GM: The development of the infra-umbilical portion of the abdominal wall, with remarks on the aetiology of ectopia vesicae. J Anat 71:201–231, 1937

Wyburn GM: Observations on the development of the human vertebral column. J Anat 78:94–102, 1944

Chapter 9

the limbs

The limbs are outgrowths of the somatopleure. They appear, towards the end of the fourth week of gestation, as thickenings of the somatic mesoderm at the level of the lower cervical and lumbar dermomyotomes. At the tip of each *limb bud* the ectodermal cells multiply to form the *apical ectodermal ridge* (Fig. 9-1).

The bud elongates by the proliferation of mesenchyme within it (Fig. 9-2). The new mesoderm arises *in situ* by mitotic activity. The greatest number of mitotic figures is found in the *progress zone* close to the apical ectodermal ridge. In the chick embryo it has been possible to mark the apical mesenchyme with carbon particles at early stages of limb development; the carbon is left behind as the limb elongates, becoming incorporated in its proximal segment. The mesenchyme of the limb segments is therefore segregated sequentially from the growing tip.

FORMATION OF HANDS AND FEET

At the end of the fifth week the primordia of the hands and feet are already apparent. They take the form of flat *limb plates,* and five mesenchymal condensations, the *digital rays,* appear in each plate (Fig. 9-3). The rays undergo chondrification and ossification to form the long bones of the hands and feet (metacarpals, metatarsals, phalanges). The apical ectodermal ridge caps the digital rays (Fig. 9-4). It ultimately forms the thick epidermis of the pad skin of fingers and toes.

The intervals between the digital rays are occupied at first by loose mesenchyme. As the digits develop these mesenchymal webs degenerate, together with the overlying ectoderm, to create the *interdigital clefts.*

LIMB SKELETON

A mesenchymal skeleton is created by cell aggregations in the core of the limb (Fig. 9-4). Chondrification centers appear in the fifth week of gestation, the whole limb skeleton being cartilaginous a week later. Ossification—or, more accurately, *osteogenesis* of the long bones

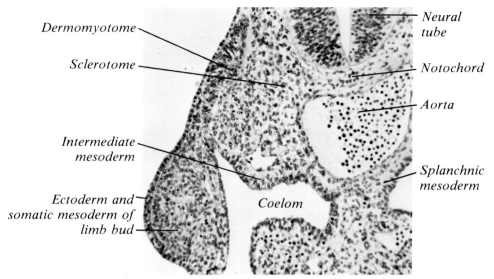

Dermomyotome

Sclerotome

Intermediate mesoderm

Ectoderm and somatic mesoderm of limb bud

Neural tube

Notochord

Aorta

Splanchnic mesoderm

Coelom

FIG. 9-1. Transverse section at upper limb bud level at four weeks' gestation. (Cambridge Collection) (x120)

FIG. 9-2. **A.** Upper limb bud at end of fifth week of gestation.
B. Enlargement from A. (Cambridge Collection) (**A**, x100; **B**, x250)

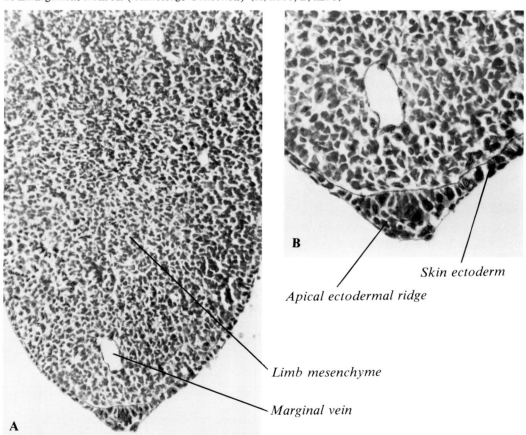

Skin ectoderm

Apical ectodermal ridge

Limb mesenchyme

Marginal vein

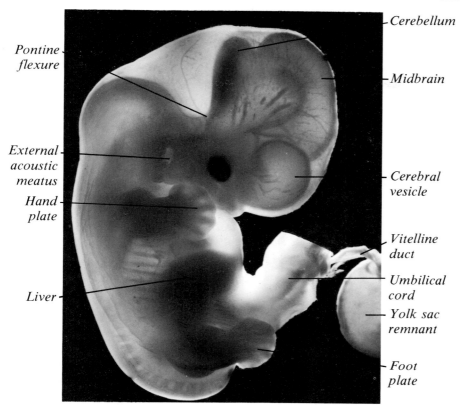

FIG. 9-3. Transilluminated six-week embryo. (x8.5)

FIG. 9-4. Skeletal elements in the upper limb at five and one-half weeks. AER, apical ectodermal ridge. (Adapted from Lewis FT, Am J Anat 2:211, 1902)

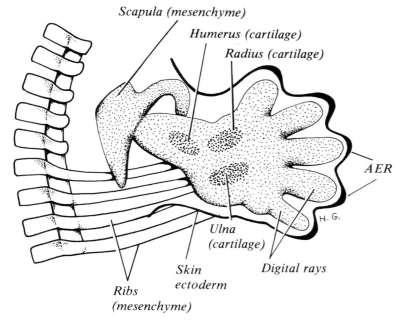

—begins in the seventh week (sixth week in the clavicle) from primary centers located in the middle of each of the cartilaginous models. It is well advanced at 12 weeks (Fig. 9-5). Ossification of the carpus begins during the first postnatal year.

For accounts of osteogenesis, the student is referred to standard textbooks of histology. The best account is probably that by Ham.

JOINTS

Where the limb cartilages articulate their perichondrium blends to form the *interzone* (Fig. 9-6A). External to the interzone, *capsular* and *synovial* thickenings differentiate from the adjacent mesenchyme. The interzone is resorbed, and clefts appear and coalesce to form the *synovial cavity* (Fig. 9-6B). The essential features of adult joint anatomy are already discernible at the beginning of the fetal period.

EXPERIMENTAL EMBRYOLOGY

In the chick, development of the limbs (wings and feet) bears a close resemblance to that of mammals. The limb buds of the chick are readily accessible for experimental procedures. Some of the more important findings are summarized in the following paragraphs.

There appears to be interplay between the apical ectodermal ridge and the progress zone. For example, if the ridge is removed from the young limb bud the proximal part of the limb grows normally but the distal limb segments fail to develop. Conversely, replacement of the

FIG. 9-5. Alizarin-stained skeleton at 12 weeks. (University of Washington Collection) (x2)

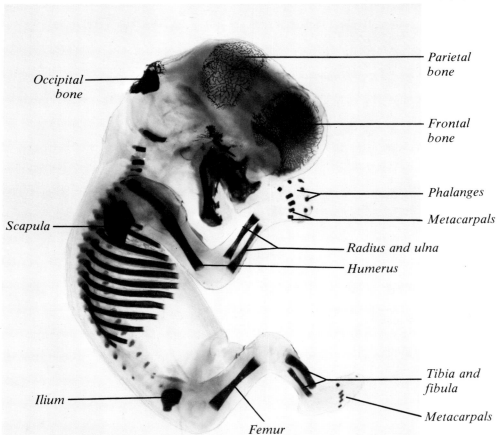

Occipital bone

Parietal bone

Frontal bone

Phalanges

Metacarpals

Radius and ulna

Humerus

Scapula

Tibia and fibula

Ilium

Metacarpals

Femur

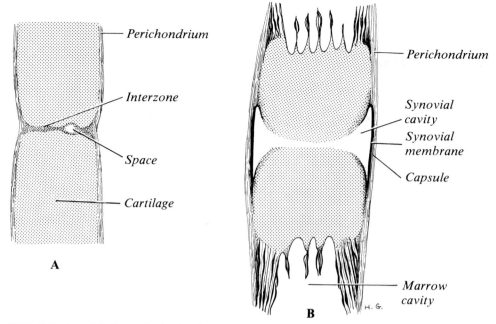

FIG. 9-6. **A** and **B.** Stages in the development of synovial joint.

progress zone by non-limb mesoderm causes the ridge to degenerate. There is evidence of inductor activity by the apical ridge upon the mesoderm, since, if the limb ectoderm is removed and two fresh ectodermal ridges are planted on the denuded mesoderm, *two sets* of digital structures develop. The main function of the apical ridge appears to be to sustain the progress zone. In man the break-up of the ridge into five parts presumably creates a progress zone for each of the digits.

As the limb bud elongates, postmitotic cells continuously leave the progress zone and differentiate sequentially to form the tissues of the appropriate segment. If the tip (progress zone plus apical ectodermal ridge) of an older limb is replaced by the tip of a young limb, then 1) the mesoderm of the older limb will form proximal (*e.g.*, thigh) structures, and 2) the young tip will add both proximal and distal structures (*e.g.*, a second thigh, and a leg and foot). The progress zone therefore appears to be autonomous, *i.e.*, uninfluenced by the degree of differentiation of the proximal part of the limb. Since the most distal parts originate from parent cells that have spent the longest time in the progress zone, all cells seem to be able to "measure" how long they have been in the zone, producing proximal or distal structures in accordance with their prior duration there. At present it is tempting to consider that the number of divisions a particular cell undergoes before release from the progress zone may determine whether the cell will differentiate into a proximal or a distal structure.

MUSCLES AND NERVES

The bulk of the musculature differentiates, *in situ,* from mesenchymal condensations on the flexor and extensor aspects of the limb cartilages. The cervical and lumbosacral myotomes probably make contributions to the girdle muscles of shoulder and hip, but microscopy offers no evidence that they migrate beyond these regions. Transplantation experiments in birds and reptiles show that in these classes at least the limb mesenchyme has muscle-forming potency.

At first the upper and lower limb buds are relatively high; the scapular condensation, for example, lies above the first rib (Fig. 9-4). They are invaded by the ventral rami of the adjacent spinal nerves (C5-T1 and L2-S3, respectively). The limbs descend during the sixth to eighth weeks, bringing the limb roots into their adult relationship.

The nerves make contact with groups of myoblasts and branch to form the brachial and lumbosacral plexuses. The motor and sensory nerve endings of the muscles (motor end-plates and muscle spindles) begin to develop during the third month. The intrafusal muscle fibers of the spindles appear to be induced by contact of *afferent* nerve fibers with the myotubules, because exclusion of sensory nerves from the developing limb prevents the development of muscle spindles. On the other hand, the development of the extrafusal muscle fibers is not dependent on the efferent innervation, since it can proceed normally in tissue culture.

The dermatomes of the limbs probably develop *in situ* beneath the skin ectoderm. They form the dermis of the skin. The cutaneous branches of the main nerve trunks supply the dermatomes in a segmental manner. There appears to be some distal migration of the dermatomes and related ectoderm over the underlying muscles, because the cutaneous territory of the mixed limb nerves is distal to the main motor territory. (The musculocutaneous, radial, femoral, and tibial nerves are the most clear-cut examples.)

ROTATION

The pollux and hallux occupy a rostral position within the limb plates. During the seventh to ninth weeks the limbs undergo *rotation* at the elbow and knee regions, to yield the adult configuration. The upper limb rotates dorsally, carrying the region of the olecranon process to the back, and the pollux to the lateral side. The lower limb rotates ventrally, carrying the future patellar region to the front, and the hallux to the medial side. Accordingly, the anterior compartments of arm and forearm are homologous with the posterior compartments of thigh and leg.

BLOOD SUPPLY

The cervical and lumbar intersegmental arteries and veins extend freely into the respective limb buds, which become permeated by anastomosing capillary networks. Preferred channels materialize; a single axial artery (seventh cervical, fifth lumbar) develops in the core of the respective limb, the blood being returned to the cardinal system by a *preaxial* vein (cephalic, great saphenous) running along the cranial border of the limb, and a *postaxial vein* (basilic, small saphenous) running along the caudal border. The early venous drainage of the upper limb is into the posterior cardinal vein, but with the descent of the heart during the second month it shifts to the anterior cardinal vein.

The developing limb skeleton displaces the axial arteries, and these arteries are largely replaced by new vessels. In the upper limb the axillary-brachial-anterior interosseous line represents the original vessel; in the lower limb the inferior gluteal artery and its sciatic branch, and the popliteal and peroneal arteries represent the original vessel (Fig. 9-7). The radial and ulnar arteries sprout from the brachial artery and take over the supply of the distal part of the upper limb. The femoral artery invades the lower limb as a new vessel; it joins the popliteal artery. The tibial arteries—new vessels homologous with the radial and ulnar—supply the leg and foot.

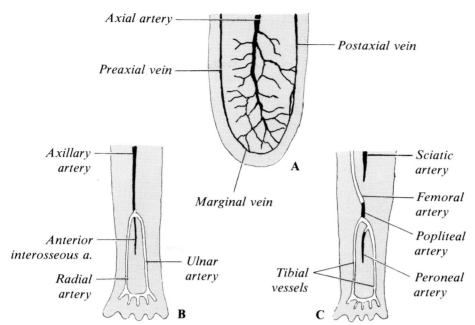

FIG. 9-7. Limb vessels: **A**, indifferent stage; **B**, upper limb; **C**, lower limb.

FIG. 9-8. The developing nail: **A**, side view; **B**, dorsal view.

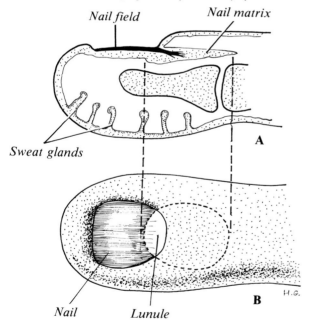

SKIN, HAIR, AND NAILS

The skin and hairs develop in the same manner as on the trunk. The *nails* are preceded by the appearance of ectodermal thickenings, the *nail fields,* on the dorsum of the terminal phalanges (tenth week). From the proximal margin of each nail field a plate of cells extends to the base of the distal phalanx. This plate is the *nail matrix,* and it includes the *lunule* (Fig. 9-8). The matrix gives rise to a thick *stratum lucidum* that extends distally, over the nail field, as the true nail. The nails reach the tips of the digits a month before term.

ABNORMALITIES

Amelia (*melos,* limb) denotes the absence of all four limbs, and *ectromelia* (*ectrome,* abortion) the absence of individual limbs. *Meromelia* denotes the partial absence of a limb; this may be *terminal, e.g.,* absence of a hand or foot, or *intercalary, e.g.,* agenesis of the radius and/or ulna, with normal development of the arm and hand.

The *lobster-claw* malformation results from complete failure of the middle digital ray. The middle metacarpal (or metatarsal) and middle digit are absent, resulting in a deep central cleft.

The degenerative process responsible for the formation of the interdigital clefts may fail either in part, with *webbing* of the affected fingers or toes, or altogether, leading to *syndactyly* (fusion of adjacent digits).

Deformities of the foot (*talipes,* or club foot) occur in as many as 1% of newborns. The great majority are examples of *postural deformity,* from compression of the feet against the wall of the uterus late in pregnancy. The normal shape of the foot is restored spontaneously after birth. Some workers draw a distinction between temporary deformities of this kind and true malformations.

SUGGESTED READING

Faber J: Vertebrate limb ontogeny and limb regeneration: morphogenetic parallels. In Abercrombie M, Brachet J, King TJ (eds): Advances in Morphogenesis, Vol 9. New York, Academic Press, 1971, pp 127–146

Frias MLM, Castilla EE, Paz JE: Descriptive system for congenital limb anomalies. Teratology 15:163–170, 1977

Goetinck PF: Genetic aspects of skin and limb development. In Mascona AA, Monroy A (eds): Current Topics in Development Biology, New York. Academic Press, 1966, pp 253–281

Ham A: The prenatal development of bone. In Histology, 7th ed. Philadelphia, JP Lippincott, 1974, pp 397–409

Kelley RO: Fine structure of the apical rim-mesenchyme complex during limb morphogenesis in man. J Embryol Exp Morphol 29:117–131, 1973

Milavie J: Aspects of limb morphogenesis in mammals. In de Haan RL, Ursprung H (eds): Organogenesis. New York, Holt, Rinehart & Winston, 1965, pp 283–300

O'Rahilly R: Morphological patterns in limb deficiencies and duplications. Am J Anat 89:135–193, 1951

Wolpert L: Mechanisms of limb development and malformations. Br Med Bull 32:65–70, 1976

Chapter 10

thoracic organs

At the end of the fourth week of gestation a *thorax* cannot yet be defined (Fig. 6-15). The heart tube is closely related to the stomodeum, to the pharynx, and to the vitelline duct. The lower respiratory tract is represented only by a median endodermal bud dorsal to the pericardium, between the thyroid and hepatic primordia. The pleural cavities are represented by the narrow pericardioperitoneal canals, and the diaphragm by the septum transversum. The body wall is formed of loose somatic mesoderm.

The thoracic cavity is formed, during the second month, by the descent of the septum transversum from the level of the middle cervical somites to that of the lower thoracic somites. The pericardioperitoneal canals elongate *pari passu*. The lungs quickly invaginate the canals, and expand to enclose the heart. The rib cage has been seen to arise by the extension of costal processes from the mesenchymal vertebrae into the somatic mesoderm.

THE HEART

In Chapter 6 it has been noted that the primitive heart tube is formed by the union of left and right endothelial channels. The *myocardium* is derived from the investment of splanchnic mesoderm.

As the heart tubes come together they display a series of dilatations, known as the *primitive heart chambers*. The most rostral chamber is the *bulbus cordis,* and the truncus arteriosus issues from it to pierce the pericardium (Fig. 10-1). The second chamber is the *ventricle*. The third is the *common atrium*. The fourth, and last to form, is the *sinus venosus*. The common atrium ascends to lie at first behind and then above the ventricle (Fig. 10-2A). It expands from side to side and embraces the truncus arteriosus. The sinus venosus receives the vitelline, umbilical, and later, the common cardinal veins. It rises within the pericardium and has left and right extensions or *horns* (Fig. 10-2B). It opens into the common atrium by the small *sinoatrial orifice.*

THE BULBOVENTRICULAR LOOP

The lengthening heart tube buckles to accommodate itself within the pericardium. The buckling is a manifestation of differential growth rather than of compression, because, in tissue culture (chick), the heart tube folds even when removed from the pericardium. A

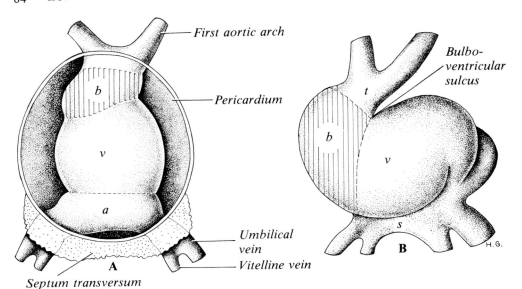

FIG. 10-1. Ventral views of the developing heart: **A**, at 21 days; **B**, at 23 days, showing the bulboventricular loop. **a**, common atrium; **b**, bulbus cordis (shaded); **s**, sinus venosus; **t**, truncus arteriosus; **v**, ventricle. (Adapted from Davis CL: Contrib Embryol Carnegie Inst 19:245–284, 1927)

FIG. 10-2. The heart at four weeks: **A**, ventral view; **B**, dorsal view. **a**, common atrium; **b**, bulbus cordis (shaded); **s**, sinus venosus; **t**, truncus arteriosus; **v**, ventricle. (Adapted from Kramer TC: Am J Anat 71:343, 1942)

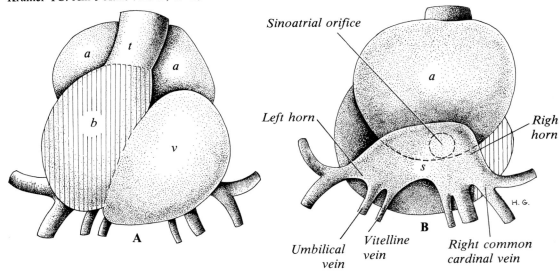

deep *bulboventricular sulcus* appears on the left side (Fig. 10-1B), and the bulbus moves to the right of the ventricle, completing the U-shaped *bulboventricular loop*.

Having invaginated the pericardium on its dorsal aspect, the primitive heart tube is initially suspended from the pericardium by the *mesocardium*. The mesocardium breaks down during the formation of the bulboventricular loop, creating the *transverse sinus* of the pericardium (Fig. 10-3). The transverse sinus can be recognized in the adult pericardial cavity as the space between the arterial and venous perforations of the pericardium.

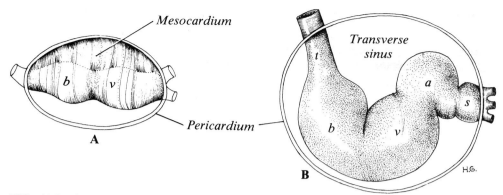

FIG. 10-3. Side views of the heart: **A,** before, **B,** following loss of the mesocardium. **a,** common atrium; **b,** bulbus cordis; **s,** sinus venosus; **t,** truncus arteriosus; **v,** ventricle.

FIG. 10-4. Scheme of the three great venous shunts (**arrows**).

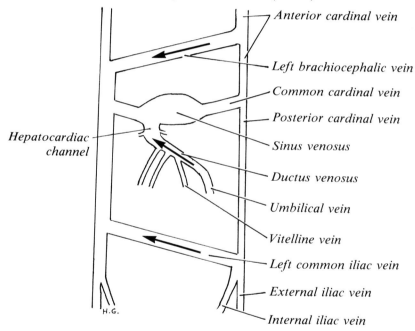

INFLUENCE OF LEFT-TO-RIGHT VENOUS SHUNTS

Three great vascular shunts divert blood from the left side of the body to the right: 1) The *left brachiocephalic vein* links the two anterior cardinal veins, and 2) the left common iliac vein links the posterior cardinal veins. The left common cardinal vein is deprived of blood by these two shunts (Fig. 10-4), and remains small. 3) The *ductus venosus* develops within the liver and receives blood from the vitelline and umbilical veins. It discharges into the right horn of the sinus venosus by the wide *hepatocardiac channel*. The left horn of the sinus venosus thereafter receives only the small input from the left common cardinal vein, and it too remains small. The increased blood flow in the right horn is accompanied by a shift of the sinoatrial orifice to the right half of the common atrium.

PARTITIONING OF THE COMMON ATRIUM

In Figure 10-5 the right wall of the common atrium has been removed. The sinoatrial orifice is seen to be guarded by the right and left *venous valves*. The atrioventricular canal is encroached upon by superior (anterior) and inferior (posterior) *endocardial cushions,* which are gelatinous subendocardial swellings.

A sickle-shaped partition, the *septum primum,* grows into the common atrium from its dorsal wall. It grows down to fuse with the endocardial cushions. Communication between left and right halves of the atrium is maintained at first by the *foramen primum* (Fig. 10-5A) at the free edge of the septum. As fusion of the septum with the cushions becomes complete, the rostral part of the septum breaks down to create the *foramen secundum* (Figs. 10-5B and 10-6).

A second sickle-shaped fold, the *septum secundum,* extends into the atrium on the right side of the septum primum (Fig. 10-5C). Its margins unite with the dorsal wall of the atrium. The interval between its free edge and the dorsal wall of the atrium is the *foramen ovale.* The foramen ovale has the septum primum in its floor (Fig. 10-5C).

THE LEFT ATRIUM

From the left half of the common atrium a vascular sprout passes back above the sinus venosus to join the plexus surrounding the developing lungs. The sprout is the embryonic *common pulmonary vein,* into which paired tributaries enter from each lung (Fig. 10-7A).

The left atrium increases in size by absorbing the pulmonary veins; at first one, then two, and finally all four veins enter it directly (Fig. 10-7C). The original, nonpulmonary component of the left atrium is represented in the adult by the trabeculated *left auricle.*

FATE OF THE SINUS VENOSUS

The right horn of the sinus venosus is incorporated into the right atrium (Fig. 10-7C). It forms the smooth-walled *sinus venarum* which receives the two caval veins and the coronary sinus. The right half of the original common atrium forms the trabeculated part of the definitive right atrium, delimited from the sinus venarum by the *crista terminalis.*

The left horn of the sinus venosus becomes the *coronary sinus* (Fig. 10-7C).

The left venous valve disappears. The right one forms the "valve" of the inferior vena cava and the valve of the coronary sinus.

FIG. 10-5. Stages in partitioning of the common atrium, viewed from the right side.

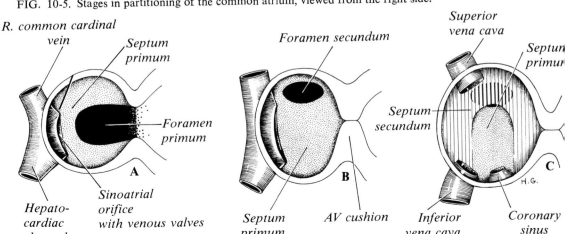

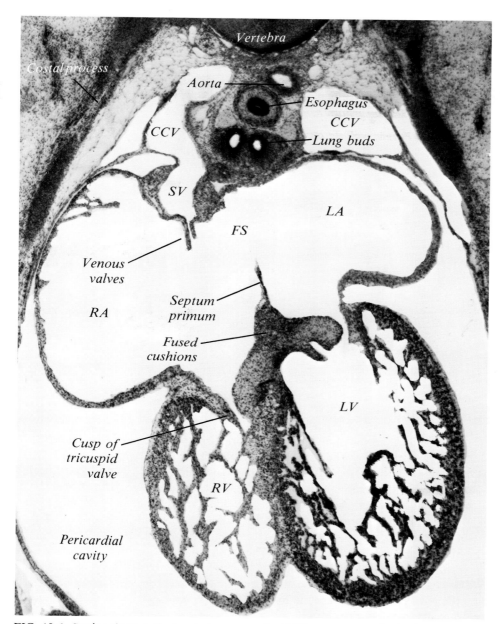

FIG. 10-6. Section through the heart at seven weeks. CCV, common cardinal vein; FS, foramen secundum; LA, left atrium; LV, left ventricle; RA, right atrium; RV, right ventricle; SV sinus venosus. (University of Washington Collection) (x100)

THE INTERATRIAL SHUNT

The function of the foramen ovale is to permit oxygenated blood to bypass the nonfunctioning fetal lungs. The fetal circulation is considered in Chapter 13, but it may be noted here that blood returning from the placenta, through the upper end of the inferior vena cava, is deflected towards the foramen ovale by the "valve" of the inferior vena cava. The septum primum yields to permit the passage of blood into the left atrium, and acts as a flap valve to prevent reflux.

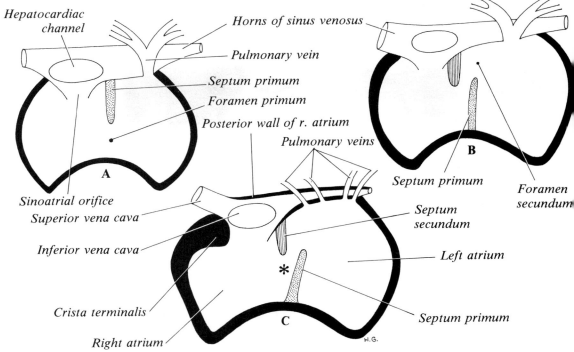

FIG. 10-7. Schematic transverse sections of the common atrium and sinus venosus. Asterisk is in foramen ovale.

THE VENTRICLES

In order to understand the terminology, it should be realized that the primitive ventricle gives rise to the *left* ventricle of the heart, and the bulbus cordis to the *right* ventricle.

The heart shown in Figure 10-8A is similar to that shown in Figure 10-1B. The ventral wall has been removed to reveal the interior of the bulboventricular loop. The atrioventricular canal is being divided by endocardial cushions into left and right channels. It opens into the ventricle. The ventricle in turn opens into the bulbus cordis. In the floor of the bulboventricular foramen a ridge—the *primitive interventricular septum*—is detectable.

Figure 10-8B corresponds to Figure 10-2A. The most significant feature is a *shift to the right, of the atrioventricular canal.* The canal has been divided by the fusion of the two atrioventricular endocardial cushions. It can be seen that the left canal opens into the ventricle and the right canal opens into the bulbus. The interventricular septum is increasing by the downward enlargement of ventricle and bulbus. The *bulboventricular ledge,* which is formed of the apposed walls of the bulboventricular sulcus, projects into the interior. The future left and right ventricles communicate through the *primary interventricular foramen,* which is bounded below by the primitive interventricular septum, above by the bulboventricular ledge, and behind by the fused atrioventricular endocardial cushions.

Next, the distal (upper) bulbus *shifts to the left,* as shown in Figure 10-9A. This shift is permitted by *absorption of the bulboventricular ledge* by the superior atrioventricular endocardial cushion so that the distal bulbus overrides the primitive interventricular septum. Both ventricles have access to the truncus arteriosus by way of the distal bulbus. The proximal bulbus forms the trabeculated part of the right ventricle. The distal bulbus forms the smooth-walled outflow portion, or *infundibulum,* of the right ventricle. It also forms the *aortic vestibule,* between the left atrioventricular orifice and the commencement of the truncus arteriosus.

The ventricles continue to deepen by the downward extension of their cavities. The

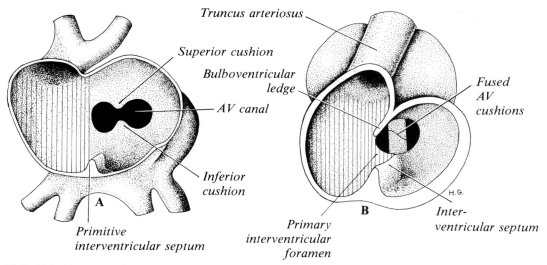

Truncus arteriosus

Superior cushion

Bulboventricular ledge

AV canal

Fused AV cushions

Inferior cushion

Primitive interventricular septum

Primary interventricular foramen

Inter-ventricular septum

FIG. 10-8. The ventricles opened from in front to show formation of the bulboventricular ledge and the rightward shift of the divided atrioventricular canal. The bulbus is shaded.

FIG. 10-9. **A.** Diagram to show the contribution of the bulbus to the ventricles. **B.** Partitioning of the outflow channel. The asterisk marks the secondary interventricular foramen.

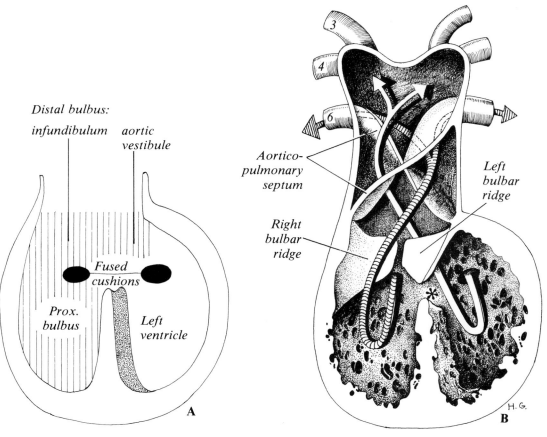

Distal bulbus:

infundibulum   aortic vestibule

Fused cushions

Prox. bulbus

Left ventricle

Aortico-pulmonary septum

Right bulbar ridge

Left bulbar ridge

atrioventricular endocardial cushions enlarge and thrust the left (future mitral) and right (future tricuspid) orifices widely apart. The dorsal part of the primitive interventricular septum fuses with the inferior cushion.

PARTITIONING OF THE OUTFLOW TRACT

The *outflow tract* of the heart comprises the distal bulbus and the truncus arteriosus. At the stage depicted in Figure 10-9A, division of the outflow tract into two streams has already begun. The division is executed by two pairs of ridges that grow into the lumen of the outflow tract. The ridges are shown in position in Figure 10-9B. The distal bulbus is divided by the left and right *bulbar ridges* composed of mesenchyme and covered with endothelium. The left ridge is attached to the left anterior wall of the distal bulbus, and the right to its right posterior wall. The two unite to form the *distal bulbar septum.* Right ventricular blood passes ventral to the distal bulbar septum to enter the anterior half of the truncus arteriosus. Left ventricular blood passes behind the septum to enter the posterior half of the truncus. For a time the ventricles communicate with one another through the *secondary interventricular foramen.* The boundaries of the secondary foramen are the same as those of the primary foramen, with the exception of its roof, which is the left part of the distal bulbar septum.

The truncus arteriosus is divided by the *aorticopulmonary septum* into *ascending aorta* and *pulmonary trunk.* This twisted septum is formed by the union of two helically disposed ridges that grow in from the walls of the truncus (Fig. 10-9B). Their disposition is probably influenced by the blood flow from the developing ventricles, the ridges developing preferentially in the relatively quiet zone between the two emerging streams. The proximal (cardiac) end of the septum is in the frontal plane, and here it fuses with the distal bulbar septum. Traced distally, the aorticopulmonary septum twists through 180 degrees. It fuses with the dorsal wall of the truncus just beyond the attachments of the sixth (pulmonary) aortic arterial arches (Fig. 10-10A).

FIG. 10-10. **A.** Partitioning of the outflow channel nearing completion in the sixth week. **B.** Definitive relationship of pulmonary vessels to the aorta.

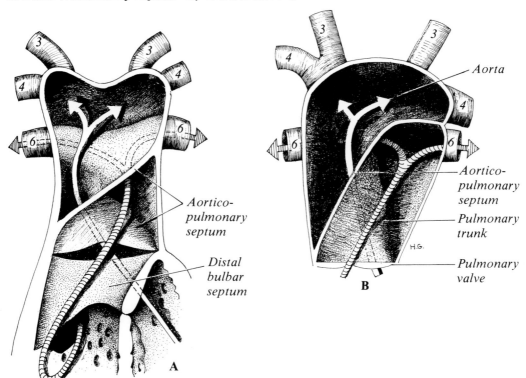

The pulmonary trunk commences in front of the aorticopulmonary septum, receiving the output from the right ventricle. It passes to the left of the aorta. The definitive trunk terminates on the left of the aorta rather than behind it; having "recruited" the two sixth arch arteries, the rostral end of the septum unwinds a little, taking the terminal part of the pulmonary trunk to the left; this movement is accompanied by elongation of the right sixth (pulmonary) artery (Fig. 10-10B).

Left ventricular blood enters the aorta dorsal to the aorticopulmonary septum. The septal torsion carries the aorta to a position ventral to the distal part of the septum. Here the aorta captures the orifices of the remaining persistent arterial arches (the third and fourth of each side).

THE HEART VALVES

The subendocardial mesenchyme forms an annular thickening around each atrioventricular orifice. The mesenchyme on the internal surface of the ventricles is excavated to create the mitral and tricuspid valves (Fig. 10-6).

The proximal end of the aorticopulmonary septum thickens at its mural attachments (Fig. 10-11A). As the aorta and pulmonary trunk begin to separate, the thickenings split to provide four of the six semilunar valves (Fig. 10-11B). Subendothelial swellings on opposite walls of the dividing truncus complete the number (Fig. 10-11C).

The left and right *coronary arteries* grow outwards above the corresponding cusps of the aortic semilunar valve.

DERIVATIVES IN THE ADULT HEART

RIGHT ATRIUM

The interatrial septum comprises the *limbus fossae ovalis,* derived from the septum secundum, and the *fossa ovalis,* a depression surrounded by the lumbus and floored by the septum primum (Fig. 10-12). The foramen ovale is sealed by adhesion of the septum primum to the limbus. The trabeculated anterior half of the atrium (including the auricle) is derived from the primitive right atrium. The smooth posterior half is derived from the right horn of the sinus venosus.

FIG. 10-11. Successive stages in development of the semilunar valves.

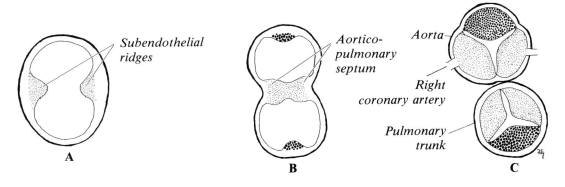

Subendothelial
ridges

Aortico-
pulmonary
septum

Aorta

Right
coronary artery

Pulmonary
trunk

A   B   C

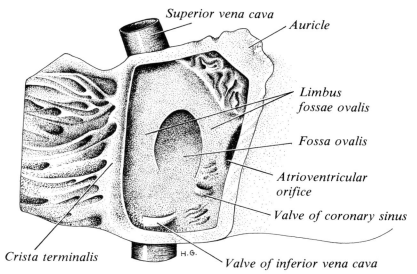

FIG. 10-12. Interior of the adult right atrium.

LEFT ATRIUM

The trabeculated left auricle appears to be the sole derivative of the primitive left atrium. The smooth atrial chamber is formed by the incorporation of the stems of the four pulmonary veins.

RIGHT VENTRICLE

The trabeculated part of the ventricle is formed by the proximal part of the bulbus cordis, and the infundibulum from the distal part (Fig. 10-13A). The lower limit of the infundibulum is marked by the *supraventricular (infundibuloventricular) crest,* which is largely formed from the right end of the distal bulbar septum.

LEFT VENTRICLE

Almost the entire left ventricle is trabeculated, and is derived from the primitive ventricle. The aortic vestibule is the smooth fibrous wall of the ventricle in the very short interval between the mitral and aortic valve rings. It is derived from the distal bulbus, whose posterior wall is so reduced here that the aortic and mitral fibrous rings come into contact (Fig. 10-13B).

INTERVENTRICULAR SEPTUM

The *lower muscular part* is formed by the primitive interventricular septum. The *upper muscular part, i.e.,* the upper anterior region, is formed by the left half of the distal bulbar septum (Fig. 10-13A). The *membranous part, i.e.,* the uppermost posterior region (Fig. 10-13B), is bounded in front by the upper muscular part, below by the lower muscular part, and behind by the ventricular wall that is formed here from inferior atrioventricular cushion tissue. It marks the site of the secondary interventricular foramen. The three boundaries mentioned may all contribute to the normal closure of the foramen, but the inferior atrioventricular cushion is usually thought to be mainly concerned.

THE GREAT VESSELS

ARTERIES

The *aortic sac* is the expanded rostral end of the truncus arteriosus. From the aortic sac five pairs of arteries (numbered 1, 2, 3, 4, and 6) pass through the branchial arches to enter the dorsal aortae. The fifth branchial arches are negligible in humans, and contain no arteries. The aortic sac is Y-shaped, having left and right *horns* from which the first four pairs of aortic arches take origin. The arteries of the sixth arch arise from the caudal, median part of the sac, which is continuous with the truncus arteriosus (Fig. 10-14A).

The first and second aortic arches regress and disappear. The third forms the stem of the *internal carotid* artery, and it gives rise to the *external carotid* artery. The segment of the dorsal aorta between the third and fourth arches on each side is lost.

The intersegmental arteries leave the dorsal aortae caudal to the sixth aortic arch. Eight are attached to the right dorsal aorta and eight to the left. More caudally they arise in pairs from the median (fused) dorsal aorta. The seventh intersegmental artery, opposite the upper limb bud, enlarges to become the *subclavian* artery (Fig. 10-14A). Vertical anastomotic channels link the subclavian to the first six intersegmentals, above, and the eighth and ninth, below: the aortic attachments of these vessels are lost. The upper vertical channel forms the *vertebral* artery, the lower one the *superior intercostal* artery (Fig. 10-14B). The third posterior intercostal artery is attached to the descending thoracic aorta, to whose upper limit it serves as a guide.

Ascent of Subclavian Arteries

The descent of the heart exerts a profound effect upon the subclavian arteries, and, as a consequence, upon the fourth aortic arches. At the end of the fifth week the heart is cranial to the limb buds and the dorsal aortae descend sharply to the level of the subclavian arteries.

FIG. 10-13. **A.** Interior of the adult right ventricle.
B. Interior of the adult left ventricle.

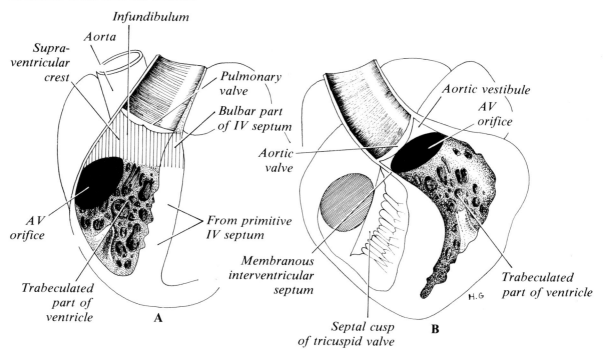

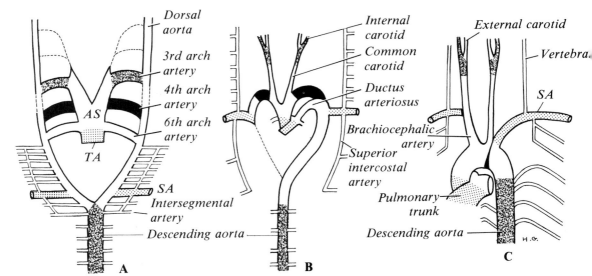

FIG. 10-14. Development of the great arteries: **A,** fifth week; **B,** seventh week; **C,** ninth week; **SA,** subclavian artery. (Adapted from Barry A: Anat Rec 111:221–238, 1951)

Two weeks later the heart and limbs are at the same level, the dorsal aortae having been "telescoped" to accommodate the change (Fig. 10-14B). After a further two weeks the heart approximates its permanent position and the subclavian vessels *ascend* to reach the roots of the limbs (Fig. 10-14C).

These changes are associated with the *virtual obliteration of the fourth aortic arch.* The subclavian artery is progressively elevated until it lies beside (left), or fuses with (right), the corresponding horn of the aortic sac. On the right side the movement is associated with attenuation and loss of the segment of the right dorsal aorta to which the eighth intersegmental artery was attached. On the left the corresponding segment remains patent to form the *left half of the arch of the definitive aorta* (Fig. 10-14C).

Fate of Aortic Sac

The right horn of the aortic sac forms the *brachiocephalic* artery and the stem of the *right common carotid* artery. The left horn forms the stem of the *left common carotid* artery. The median, unpaired portion forms the *right half of the arch of the definitive aorta* (Fig. 10-14C).

Sixth Aortic Arch

As the arteries of the sixth arch grow dorsally from the aortic sac, they are diverted to the lung buds and become the primitive *pulmonary arteries.* The arterial arches are completed by a ventral extension from each dorsal aorta.

On the right side the distal portion of the sixth artery is lost. On the left the distal portion becomes the *ductus arteriosus.* The function of the ductus is to act as a pulmonary bypass. Before birth the lungs receive only sufficient blood to establish a pulmonary vascular bed in preparation for respiratory activity; the rest is shunted to the placenta by way of the ductus arteriosus and the descending aorta.

The development of the great arteries is summarized in Table 10-1.

TABLE 10-1. ORIGINS OF THE GREAT ARTERIES

ARTERY	ORIGIN
Pulmonary trunk	Truncus arteriosus
Pulmonary arteries	Sixth arch arteries
Aortic arch, right half	Aortic sac
Aortic arch, left half	Left dorsal aorta
Brachiocephalic	Aortic sac
Common carotids	Aortic sac
Internal carotids	Third arch arteries, and cranial extensions of dorsal aortae
External carotids	From third arch arteries
Subclavians	Seventh intersegmental arteries

VEINS

The symmetry of the cardinal venous system is broken by the left brachiocephalic vein, which diverts blood from the left to the right anterior cardinal vein (Fig. 10-15A and B). The posterior cardinal system of both sides is almost entirely replaced during the construction of the inferior vena cava, and a new, *azygos,* system drains the intercostal spaces. Despite its name (*azygos,* unpaired), this is a symmetrical system at first; later, however, two cross-channels divide the left main vessel into hemiazygos and accessory hemiazygos veins, and drain into the (right) azygos trunk (Fig. 10-15C).

Upon the entry of the main (subclavian) limb veins into the anterior cardinals, the cranial portions of the anterior cardinals are termed the *internal jugular veins* (Fig. 10-15C).

FIG. 10-15. Stages in development of the intrathoracic veins.

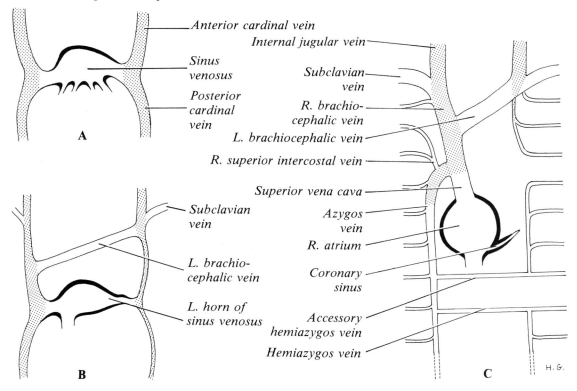

Each internal jugular joins the corresponding subclavian to form a brachiocephalic vein, and these veins meet to form the cranial part of the *superior vena cava*. The upper end of the right posterior cardinal vein persists as the *arch of the azygos vein*. The right common cardinal vein forms the lower part of the superior vena cava. The left posterior and common cardinal veins, deprived of blood by the right-to-left shunts, dwindle to become the *left superior intercostal vein* and the *oblique vein of left atrium* respectively.

HEMOPOIESIS

The development of the cells of the blood may be conveniently considered here. The first cells to form are the nucleated *hemocytoblasts,* which are found in the blood islands of the yolk sac during the third week of gestation (Fig. 6-11). They develop from the extraembryonic mesoderm. Tissue culture experiments (in mice) indicate that the yolk sac hemocytoblasts are the precursors of all the cells of the erythroid series, and that other stem cells of the yolk sac give rise to all the white cells.

Hemocytoblasts leave the yolk sac to enter the circulation early in the fourth week. They multiply within the circulation to form the *primitive erythroblasts*—nucleated red blood cells which persist through the 12th week. *Definitive erythropoiesis,* leading to the production of nonnucleated erythrocytes, commences in the liver during the sixth week. The "hepatic period" of erythropoiesis is shared to a small extent by the spleen and reaches its peak at about the 16th week. It tapers off in later fetal life and terminates at about the time of birth (Fig. 10-16).

Hemopoiesis in the bone marrow begins at about week 16 and increases progressively. After birth the bone marrow is normally the only site of red-cell production.

White blood cells (granulocytes) appear to develop from stem cells that migrate from the yolk sac to the bone marrow. Mature granulocytes enter the circulation from the marrow during and after the tenth week.

Lymphocyte development commences in the thymus (see section "Thymus" in Chapter 12) in the ninth week of gestation and in lymph nodes about a week later. Mature lymphocytes are found in the blood after the tenth week.

FIG. 10-16. Successive stages in erythropoiesis. (Adapted from Wintrobe MW, et al.: Clinical Hematology, 7th ed. Philadelphia, Lea & Febiger, 1974, pp 41–79)

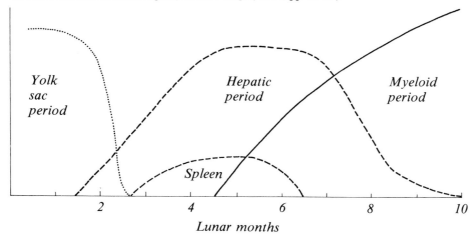

LUNGS, PLEURA, DIAPHRAGM

Three stages in the history of the embryonic coelom have already been described. They were 1) the appearance of a U-shaped cleft in the embryonic mesoderm; 2) flexion of the rostral part of the coelom (*i.e.,* the pericardial cavity) during the formation of the head fold; 3) union of the caudal parts of the coelom around the vitellointestinal duct during lateral flexion, creating the peritoneal cavity. The paired passages linking the pericardial and peritoneal cavities are the pericardioperitoneal canals, or *coelomic ducts* (Fig. 10-17).

LUNGS AND PLEURA

The lower respiratory system is an outgrowth of the foregut. It appears in the fourth week of gestation as a median diverticulum in its floor (Fig. 6-16). In the fifth week the respiratory diverticulum divides into two *lung buds* which invaginate the respective pericardioperitoneal canals from their dorsomedial aspect. The canals are then called the *pleural cavities.*

The connection of each pleural cavity with the pericardial sac is reduced by the *pleuropericardial membrane,* a mesodermal fold lodging the common cardinal vein (Fig. 10-17). The communication with the peritoneal cavity is reduced by the *pleuroperitoneal membrane,* a sickle-shaped ingrowth of the somatic mesoderm opposite the septum transversum.

The primitive esophagus extends from the point of origin of the respiratory diverticulum to the dorsal edge of the septum transversum. It is very short, lying entirely behind the heart (Fig. 10-18A). The pharyngeal arches gain the midline by insinuation between the foregut and the pericardium, causing progressive caudal displacement of the heart and of the septum transversum (on which the heart lies). The vitelline duct, straddled by the septum

FIG. 10-17. Ventral view of the pericardial cavity following removal of the heart at five weeks' gestation. The opening of the coelomic duct is seen on each side. The trachea and lung buds lie behind the pericardium. (Adapted from Wells LJ: Contrib Embryol Carnegie Inst 35:107–134, 1954)

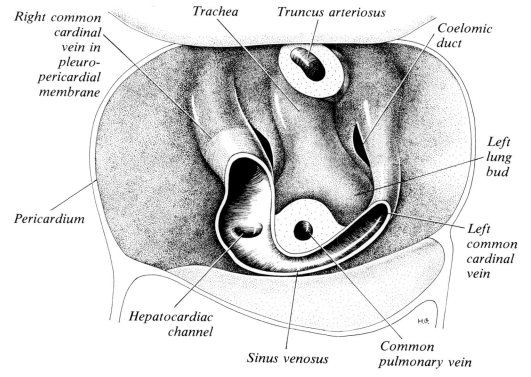

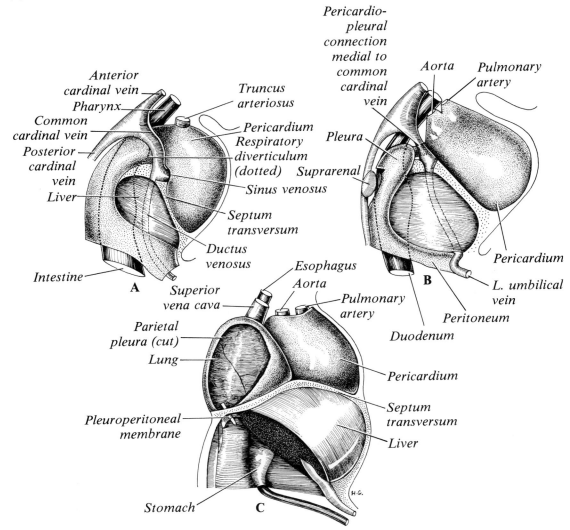

FIG. 10-18. Side views of the embryonic coelom: **A**, at four weeks; **B**, during the sixth week; **C**, at seven weeks, with a "rod" in the pleuroperitoneal canal. (A and B adapted from Wells LJ: Contrib Embryol Carnegie Inst 35:107–134, 1954; C adapted from Bleckschmidt E: The Stages of Human Development before Birth. Philadelphia, WB Saunders, 1961, p 515)

transversum, is displaced in turn; this aids the closure of the duct. Descent of the heart is arrested late in the second month by the prodigious growth of the liver. The heart is then enclosed, together with the lungs, in the cage formed by the developing ribs.

The fourth and sixth branchial arches give rise to the cartilages and muscles of the larynx, and to the constrictor muscles which invest the foregut from the oral cavity to the level of the cricoid cartilage. The segment of primitive esophagus behind the larynx is called the *laryngeal pharynx;* the *definitive esophagus* commences at the lower edge of the inferior contrictor.

Cardiac descent imposes an increasing obliquity on the common cardinal veins. The covering pleuropericardial membrane is drawn medially, and it fuses with the wall of the esophagus, thereby separating pleura from pericardium (Fig. 10-18B).

The pleuroperitoneal membranes descend opposite the septum transversum, thereby lengthening the pleural cavities. They blend with the septum at the end of the seventh week, to seal off the pleural sacs. The septum and membranes are shelflike, and their successful union demands the support of the liver below the septum, and of the suprarenal glands below the membranes. Failure of closure of the pleuroperitoneal orifice, when it occurs, tends to be left-sided; this is attributable to the greater bulk of the liver's right lobe than of its left lobe.

The medial surfaces of the pleural cavities invest the lung buds, forming the *visceral pleura*. The lung buds increase in size by repeated division of each main stem. They quickly outgrow the pleural cavities and begin to excavate the somatic mesoderm along the line of attachment of the pleuroperitoneal folds. The lungs extend almost to the midline before and behind the heart by peeling off a "rind" of somatic mesoderm. They pass dorsal to the esophagus, creating a *retroesophageal septum* between esophagus and aorta. Finally, they expand upwards, ballooning into the body wall lateral to the cardinal veins. In this way the superior vena cava and azygos vein come to lie medial to the upper lobe of the right lung (Fig. 10-18C).

Blood Supply of the Lungs

The respiratory diverticulum and embryonic foregut are surrounded by a vascular plexus fed by twigs from the dorsal aorta. The plexus drains into the adjacent cardinal veins. Each lung bud, as it enters the coelomic duct, induces a side sprout—the *pulmonary artery*—from the corresponding sixth aortic arch; the blood supply from the dorsal aorta is reduced to one or two *bronchial arteries*. The venous drainage is captured in turn by the common pulmonary vein, and the connection with the cardinal system is lost.

Histogenesis of the Lungs

The left lung bud divides into two and the right into three branches; these later become canalized to form the *main* and *lobar bronchi*. From the lobar bronchi arise the segmental

FIG. 10-19. The lung buds.
A. Transverse section at five weeks. CCV, common cardinal vein. (Carnegie Collection) (x60)
B. Parasagittal section at six weeks. HC, hepatocardiac channel; TA, truncus arteriosus.
(Cambridge Collection) (x40)

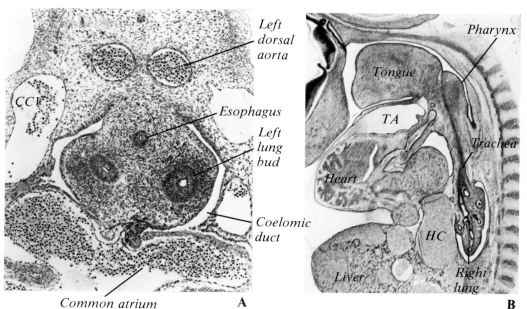

branches, which ultimately form the wedge-shaped *bronchopulmonary segments* that are present in the adult.

The endodermal buds carry with them an investment of splanchnic mesoderm (Fig. 10-19). Both endoderm and mesoderm differentiate proximodistally, the former giving rise to the respiratory epithelium and the latter to the tracheobronchial cartilages and musculature. Organ culture studies indicate that the mesoderm investing the bronchial buds induces the buds' progressive branching. The buds fail to branch when separated from the specific (bronchial) mesoderm.

During the fifth month of gestation the lungs resemble an exocrine gland, the bronchial subdivisions ending in *alveolar sacs* lined by cubical epithelium. Alveolar development sets in during the fifth month; it is characterized by prolific multiplication of the pulmonary capillaries around the terminal (bronchiolar) buds, whose endoderm thins out to form flattened *alveolar cells* in close relationship to the vessels. The individual alveoli are poorly developed at birth, and the physiologic unit of the lung is probably the alveolar sac.

During the first five postnatal years the number of alveoli shows a tenfold increase. Branching of the respiratory tree, however, ceases about the time of birth; the new alveoli evidently arise from the continued differentiation of the terminal buds, so that terminal branchioles become converted into respiratory bronchioles and respiratory bronchioles into alveolar ducts (Fig. 10-20).

DIAPHRAGM

The diaphragm has the following components (Fig. 10-21):

1. The septum transversum, which gives rise to the central tendon.
2. The retroesophageal septum, which contributes connective tissue to the posterior median part.
3. The pleuroperitoneal membranes.
4. The rim of excavated body-wall mesoderm.
5. Cervical myotomes. The pleuroperitoneal membranes, when first seen, are at the level of the third to fifth cervical myotomes. From these myotomes, premuscle cells are believed to enter the membranes, to form the musculature of the diaphragm. The ventral rami of the corresponding spinal nerves make up the phrenic nerve. The myotomes become

FIG. 10-20. Changing structure of the bronchial tree: **A**, newborn; **B**, child about two years old. (Respiratory bronchioles have some alveoli in their walls. Alveolar ducts lead to alveolar sacs, each of which is lined [B] by a cluster of alveoli.)

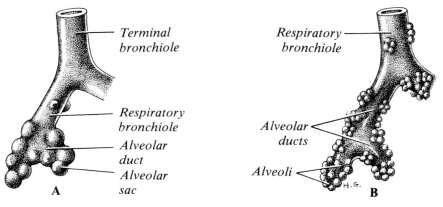

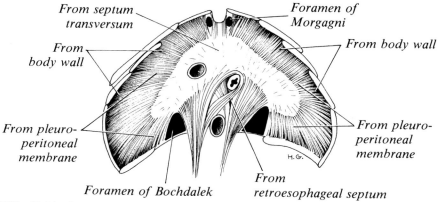

From septum transversum

Foramen of Morgagni

From body wall

From body wall

From pleuro-peritoneal membrane

From pleuro-peritoneal membrane

H.G.

Foramen of Bochdalek

From retroesophageal septum

FIG. 10-21. Component parts of the diaphragm.

attached to the lower six ribs and to the upper lumbar vertebrae. In man the phrenic nerve is entirely responsible for the motor supply to the diaphragm, and it is also sensory to the serous membranes on its upper and lower surfaces. The lower six intercostal nerves are sensory to the pleura close to the costal attachments of the diaphragm.

THORACIC DUCT

The thoracic duct is the chief lymphatic vessel. It conveys the lymph from three quadrants of the body to the general circulation. From the fourth quadrant (right side of thorax, right upper limb, and right side of head and neck) the lymph enters the circulation through the right lymphatic duct.

All the lymphatic vessels grow out from the *primary lymph sacs,* which are arranged as follows: 1) a pair of *jugular sacs* at the root of the neck, 2) a pair of *iliac sacs* in the lower abdomen, 3) a *retroperitoneal sac* at the root of the mesentery of the intestine, and 4) the *cisterna chyli,* below the diaphragm. From the sacs, lymphatic vesesls grow along the main veins of the head, neck, limbs, and abdomen.

The cisterna chyli is linked to the two jugular sacs by a left and a right thoracic lymph vessel. The *thoracic duct* is derived from the lower part of the right duct and the upper part of the left; an oblique channel crosses the midline behind the esophagus to establish the linkage. The upper part of the right thoracic lymph vessel persists as the *right lymphatic duct.*

ABNORMALITIES

THE HEART

Recognized cardiac malformations, occurring alone or in combination, number more than one hundred. Only brief comments are warranted here.

Malformations are potentially dangerous in two ways: 1) They may permit an *arteriovenous shunt* between right and left sides of the heart. Sufficient blood may bypass the lungs to cause cyanosis from poor oxygen saturation (the so-called "blue baby"). 2) One of the heart channels may be so narrowed as to cause congestive heart failure or to render the endocardium susceptible to blood-borne infection.

About 50% of all cases fall into the following four categories, listed in order of incidence: *isolated ventricular septal defect, isolated atrial septal defect, tetralogy of Fallot, and isolated pulmonary stenosis.* These conditions are amenable to surgery.

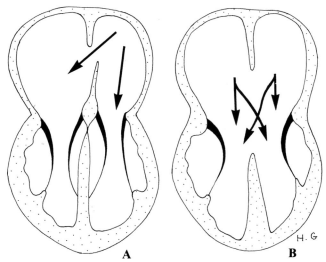

FIG. 10-22. Atrial septal defects: **A,** patent foramen ovale; **B,** persistent foramen primum. **Arrows** indicate direction of blood flow.

Atrial Septal Defect

Isolated atrial septal defect almost always takes the form of a *patent foramen ovale*. Minor communication through the foramen ("probe patency") is found in about 25% of adults and is without significance. A major defect causes an arteriovenous shunt (Fig. 10-22A). The fault lies in an unduly large foramen secundum.

Rarely the defect is due to a persistent foramen primum. In this condition there is evidence of growth failure in the region of the atrioventricular canal; the upper part of the interventricular septum and the septal cusps of the atrioventricular valves are also deficient (Fig. 10-22B).

Isolated Ventricular Septal Defect

The junctional nature of the membranous part of the interventricular septum renders this region especially liable to faulty development, and it is here that a ventricular septal defect is usually found. As a rule, ventricular blood is shunted from left to right (Fig. 10-23A).

Isolated Pulmonary Stenosis

Narrowing of the pulmonary channel may be infundibular, valvular, or supravalvular. In infundibular stenosis the distal bulbus is regarded as having been abnormally small (Fig. 10-23B). In the other two forms the aorticopulmonary septum is thought to have been laid down "off center," the pulmonary section of the divided truncus arteriosus being relatively narrow.

Fallot's Tetralogy

The syndrome comprises 1) infundibular pulmonary stenosis, 2) hypertrophy of the right ventricle, as a result of the stenosis, 3) an overriding aorta that communicates with both ventricles, and 4) a high ventricular septal defect (Fig. 10-23C). The primary fault appears to lie in the embryonic bulbus; the normal leftward shift of the bulbus is incomplete, so that the aorta is not brought into full communication with the left ventricle, and (perhaps

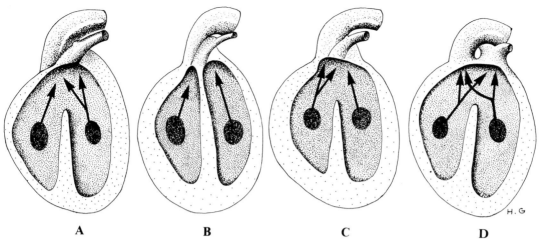

FIG. 10-23. Malformations of the outflow tracts. **A**, isolated ventricular septal defect; **B**, isolated pulmonary stenosis; **C**, Fallot's tetralogy; **D**, transposition of great vessels.

because of this) the distal bulbar septum is too ventrally placed, reducing the size of the infundibulum. Fallot's tetralogy is the commonest cause of cyanotic heart disease.

Transposition of the Great Vessels

The aorta arises from the right ventricle and the pulmonary trunk from the left (Fig. 10-23D). The aorticopulmonary system must have been straight, and in the sagittal plane, to account for the final relationships. However, the straight septum may have been caused by altered blood flow in the truncus becouse of malposition of the distal bulbar septum.

Abnormal Positions of the Heart

Situs inversus viscerum is characterized by reversal of the normal position of the viscera— the heart, stomach, and spleen are right-sided and the liver and appendix are on the left. Total situs inversus is not a cause for concern, but if the heart *alone* is left-sided (*isolated levocardia*) it is always malformed.

GREAT VESSELS

Patent Ductus Arteriosus

The ductus arteriosus normally undergoes rapid closure after birth, shrinking to become a fibrous cord—the *ligamentum arteriosum*. Failure of closure allows an extensive leakage into the pulmonary circulation from the aorta, with corresponding impairment of circulatory efficiency. Patent ductus arteriosus accounts for 10% of cardiovascular malformations.

Coarctation of the Aorta

In coarctation (*arctare,* to tighten) the aorta is occluded in the region of attachment of the ligamentum arteriosum (Fig. 10-24A). For 1 cm or more, the vessel may be replaced by a fibrous cord. The blood supply to the lower part of the body is maintained by the collateral vessels that link the subclavian arteries to the descending aorta and its branches. The

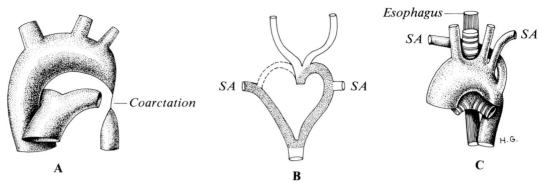

FIG. 10-24. **A.** Coarctation of the aorta.
B. Embryonic.
C. Adult arrangement in anomalous right subclavian artery (SA).

occlusion is probably the result of involvement of the aorta in the histologic processes concerned in closure of the ductus arteriosus.

Malformations of Aortic Arch

The components of the definitive arch may develop on the right side instead of the left, the aorta passing to the right side of the trachea and esophagus. Rarely, development is symmetrical and a *double aortic arch* may compress trachea and esophagus. Persistence of the right dorsal aorta distal to the subclavian artery results in the curious *anomalous right subclavian artery* (Fig. 10-24B and C).

LUNGS

A common anomaly (0.5% of the population) is the so-called *azygos lobe,* created by expansion of the right upper lobe on *both* sides of the posterior cardinal (azygos) vein. The radiologic appearance provides the diagnosis.

    Agenesis of a lung, or of a pulmonary lobe, is rare. *Pulmonary isomerism* follows enantiomorphic (mirror-image) division of the trachea, the right lung acquiring two lobes and the left three. *Congenital cysts* of the lung are lined by ciliated epithelium and they communicate with the bronchial tree.

DIAPHRAGM

Herniation of abdominal contents through the diaphragm is common. It can be demonstrated radiologically in about 2% of radiologic studies of the upper gastrointestinal tract. In 80% of its subjects the hernia occupies the esophageal hiatus in the diaphragm (so-called *hiatus hernia*). Most hiatus hernias first appear in adult life, but they are probably due to congenital weakness of this part of the diaphragm. In *congenital short esophagus,* part or all of the stomach lies in the posterior mediastinum, where it receives its blood supply directly from the thoracic aorta.

    The pleuroperitoneal communication may persist (on the left side, as a rule) as the *foramen of Bochdalek* (Fig. 10-21), through which extensive congenital herniation of abdominal viscera may occur. The rare *foramen of Morgagni* is a congenital gap between sternal and costal origins of the diaphragm; it permits herniation to take place into the anterior mediastinum (Fig. 10-21).

    Congenital eventration of the diaphragm results from failure of development of the phrenic musculature on one side. The affected dome is pushed up by the abdominal viscera, and rides high in the chest.

SUGGESTED READING

Anderson RH, Wilkinson JL, Arnold R: Morphogenesis of bulboventricular malformations. 1. Consideration of embryogenesis in the normal heart. Br Heart J 36:242–255, 1974

Barry A: Aortic arch derivatives in the human adult. Anat Rec 111:221–238, 1951

Boyden EA: Development of the human lung. In Brennemann's Practice of Pediatrics, Vol 4. Hagerstown, Harper & Row, 1972, pp 1–12

De Haan RL: Development of form in the embryonic heart. Circulation 35:821–833, 1967

Goor DA, Dische R, Lillehei CW: The conotruncus. 1. Its normal inversion and conus absorption. Circulation 46:375–389, 1972

Goor DA, Edwards JE, Lillehei CW: The development of the interventricular septum of the normal heart; correlative morphogenetic study. Chest 58:453–467, 1970

Spooner BS, Wessells NK: Mammalian lung development: interactions in primordium formation and bronchial morphogenesis. J Exp Zool 175:445–454, 1970

Wells LJ: Development of the human diaphragm and pleural sac. Contrib Embryol Carnegie Inst 35:107–134, 1954

Wintrobe MW, Lee GR, Boggs DR, Bithall TC, Athens JW, Foerster J: Origin and development of the blood and blood-forming tissues. In Clinical Hematology, 7th ed. Philadelphia, Lea & Febiger, 1974, pp 41–79

Chapter 11

abdominal and pelvic organs

Before the end of the fourth week of gestation the head and tail folds have progressed sufficiently to define the embryonic foregut, midgut, and hindgut (Fig. 6-15). The midgut faces the yolk sac remnant through a wide vitelline duct. The embryonic and extraembryonic parts of the coelom are in communication beside the midgut. Cranially, the embryonic coelom leads to the pericardial cavity, and it has blind caudal (pelvic) extensions.

The septum transversum intervenes between midgut and pericardium. The hepatic primordium is a median thickening of the endoderm in contact with the septum. Close by, the vitelline and umbilical veins pass through the septum to enter the sinus venosus.

Growth of the mesoderm outpaces that of the endoderm, and the gut undergoes a relative reduction in size. Completion of lateral flexion reduces the umbilical opening of the embryonic coelom (Fig. 8-12). Cranial and caudal to the dwindling vitelline duct, the left and right coelomic ducts join to form the peritoneal cavity. Dorsal to the gut the coelom approaches the midline so that the gut is suspended by a dorsal mesentery (Fig. 11-1).

Cranial to the hepatic primordium the foregut expands to form the *stomach*. The coelom, extending ventral to the stomach, encounters the septum transversum and encroaches on it from either side to create the so-called *ventral mesentery* of the foregut, which is in fact a septum, not a mesentery. Ventrally, the ventral mesentry is attached to the somatopleure of the abdominal wall; rostrally to the shelflike part of the septum transversum in contact with the pericardium; and, dorsally, to the stomach and duodenum as far as the origin of the hepatic primordium. Its caudal edge is free (Fig. 11-2).

The right and left vitelline veins run on the corresponding surfaces of the vitelline duct and foregut. They pass through the ventral mesentery to reach the heart. The umbilical veins, at first lateral to the coelom, are carried ventrally in the somatopleure (Fig. 11-1) to be incorporated in the ventral attachment of the mesentery.

LIVER AND GALLBLADDER

The cells of the hepatic diverticulum (Fig. 11-3) penetrate the loose mesenchyme of the ventral mesentery and divide into ventral and dorsal cell buds. The ventral bud stays close to the free edge of the mesentery, and acquires a lumen to become the primitive *gallbladder*. The dorsal bud divides in turn into left and right *liver lobe primordia,* and these multiply to form an epithelial spongework which taps first the vitelline and then the umbilical veins.

106

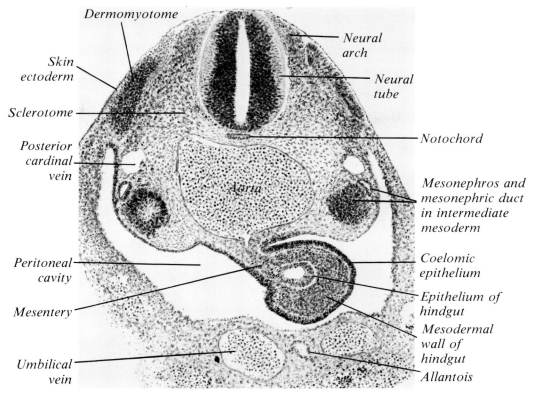

Dermomyotome

Skin ectoderm

Sclerotome

Posterior cardinal vein

Peritoneal cavity

Mesentery

Umbilical vein

Neural arch

Neural tube

Notochord

Aorta

Mesonephros and mesonephric duct in intermediate mesoderm

Coelomic epithelium

Epithelium of hindgut

Mesodermal wall of hindgut

Allantois

FIG. 11-1. Transverse section through the caudal part of a four-week embryo. (Carnegie Collection) (x80)

FIG. 11-2. Diagram of the dorsal and ventral mesenteries of the gut.

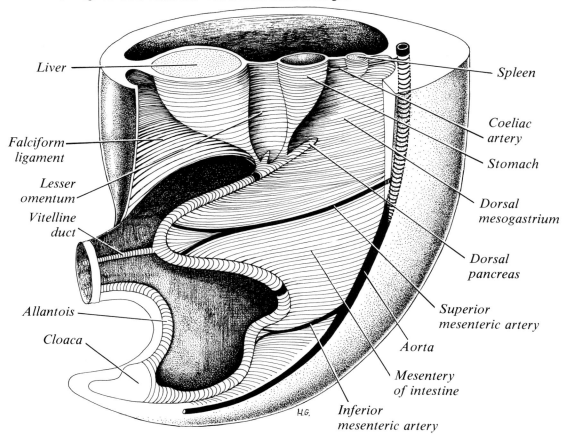

Liver

Falciform ligament

Lesser omentum

Vitelline duct

Allantois

Cloaca

Spleen

Coeliac artery

Stomach

Dorsal mesogastrium

Dorsal pancreas

Superior mesenteric artery

Aorta

Mesentery of intestine

Inferior mesenteric artery

H.G.

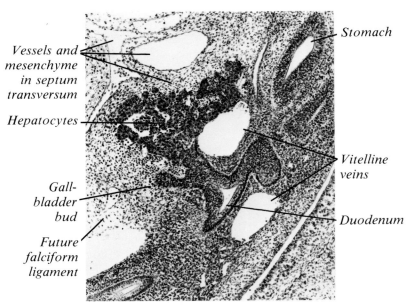

FIG. 11-3. Sagittal section through the hepatic bud at three and one-half weeks' gestation. (Carnegie Collection) (x60)

The liver epithelium is later organized around radicles of the vitelline veins in the form of ill-defined *lobules*. The stem of the hepatic primordium becomes the *bile duct*. The connection of the ventral bud to it forms the *cystic duct,* and the divisions of the dorsal bud become the *left* and *right hepatic ducts* (Fig. 11-13).

Under the influence of the surrounding mesoderm, the liver epithelium differentiates into *hepatocytes*. The vitelline endothelial cells acquire a phagocytic function to become *Kupffer cells*. The bulk of the liver is increased by the appearance within it of blood islands, where hemopoiesis increases until the third month, at which time the organ makes up 10% of the body weight. Blood formation in the liver decreases during pregnancy and ceases at full term. However, it may be resumed during postnatal life in certain pathologic states.

The liver expands into the coelomic cavity, dividing the ventral mesentery into the *falciform ligament,* which extends from the liver to the abdominal wall, and the *lesser omentum,* which passes from the liver to the foregut (Fig. 11-2). The mesoderm of the mesentery also contributes to the connective tissue of the liver (Glisson's capsule).

Cephalic extension of the liver brings it into contact with the upper, horizontal part of the septum transversum as this differentiates to form the central part of the diaphragm. The "bare area" of the liver is created by enlargement of the region of direct contact with the diaphragm (Fig. 11-4A). Side-to-side expansion gives rise to the right and left *triangular ligaments;* dorsal expansion brings the "bare area" into contact with the inferior vena cava and with the right suprarenal gland and kidney (Fig. 11-4B).

TRANSFORMATION OF THE VITELLINE AND UMBILICAL VEINS

The impact of the liver upon the vitelline and umbilical veins produces radical changes in their disposition. The sequence of events is as follows (Fig. 11-5):

1. As they enter the ventral mesentery from below, the vitelline veins (**A**) fuse to become the terminal segment of the *portal vein.* Cranial to this, they are then its left and right branches (**B**).
2. The vitelline veins are disrupted in the center of each primitive liver lobe (**C**).

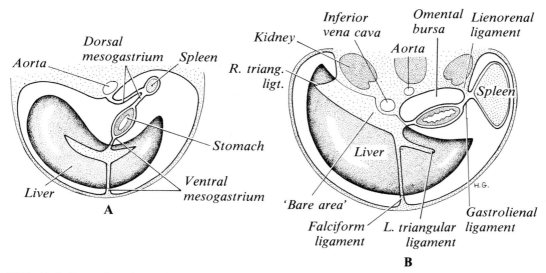

FIG. 11-4. Formation of the triangular ligaments and the "bare area" of the liver, and omental bursa, viewed from above.

FIG. 11-5. Transformation of the vitelline and umbilical veins.

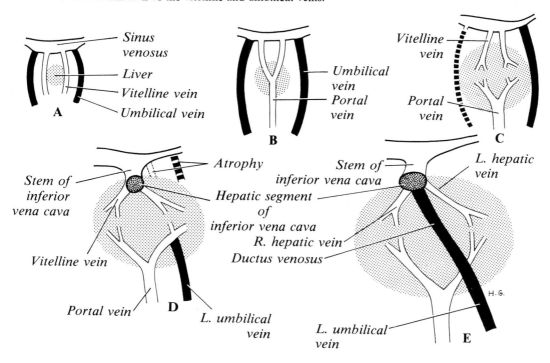

3. The number of vitelline and umbilical veins entering the sinus venosus is reduced from four to one by a succession of intricate changes in blood flow:
   (a) The right vitelline vein, where it leaves the liver, expands to form the *hepatocardiac channel.*
   (b) The inferior vena cava, whose history is described later in this chapter, enters the hepatocardiac channel from its dorsal aspect, and the channel is thereafter called the *stem of the inferior vena cava* (**C**).

(c) The terminal part of the left vitelline vein is lost (**D**). The veins draining the left lobe open into the stem of the inferior vena cava by a new channel, the *left hepatic vein*. The right vitelline vein immediately caudal to the entry of the inferior vena cava is now termed the *right hepatic vein* (**E**).

(d) The liver trabeculae, expanding in all directions, invade the umbilical veins. The right umbilical vein atrophies throughout its entire extent, leaving no trace (**C**). *The left umbilical vein then carries all the oxygenated blood from the placenta to the embryo.* It meets the left branch of the portal vein within the liver (**D**).

(e) A wide, intrahepatic space appears between the left umbilical vein and the hepato-cardiac channel. This is the *ductus venosus* (**E**), which sweeps the placental blood through to the heart by the most direct route (Fig. 11-6). The terminal segment of the left umbilical vein, deprived of blood by the ductus venosus, disappears (**D**).

The circulatory changes at birth are considered in Chapter 13. Here it is relevant to note the fate of the umbilical venous pathway after the cessation of blood flow through it at birth. The left umbilical vein shrinks to become the *ligamentum teres* in the free edge of the falciform ligament, extending from the umbilicus to the left branch of the portal vein. The ductus venosus becomes the fibrous *ligamentum venosum,* stretching from the latter point to the stem of the inferior vena cava.

STOMACH AND OMENTAL BURSA

During the fifth and sixth weeks of gestation the stomach appears to undergo rotation through 90 degrees (Figs. 11-4 and 11-7). The line of attachment of the ventral mesogas-trium moves to the right, and that of the dorsal mesogastrium to the left. The peritoneal recess that lies behind the stomach, and extends into the dorsal mesentery, is the *omental bursa* (lesser sac of peritoneum). The stomach is flattened dorsoventrally, displaying anterior and posterior surfaces. To what extent there is genuine rotation of the stomach is

FIG. 11-6. Sagittal section at 10 weeks, showing the ductus venosus. (Carnegie Collection) (x14)

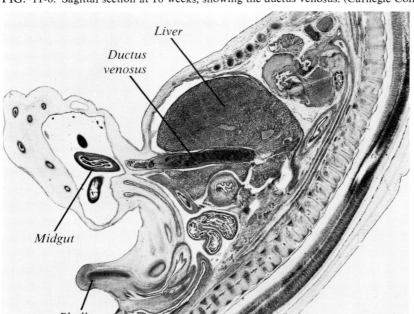

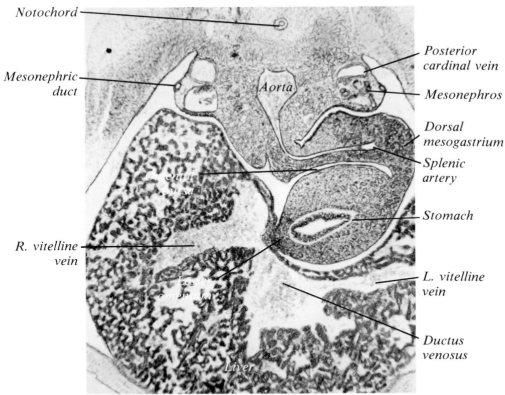

Notochord

Mesonephric duct

Aorta

Posterior cardinal vein

Mesonephros

Dorsal mesogastrium

Splenic artery

Stomach

R. vitelline vein

L. vitelline vein

Ductus venosus

Liver

FIG. 11-7. Transverse section of upper abdominal organs early in the sixth week of gestation. (Carnegie Collection) (x12)

uncertain. (The disposition of the *gastric nerves* in the adult is adduced as evidence of gastric rotation, because the anterior gastric nerve is derived mainly from the left vagus and the posterior gastric mainly from the right vagus. Contrary to some descriptions, inspection of the longitudinal muscle coat of the esophagus offers no evidence that gastric "rotation" twists the lower end of the esophagus. However, differentiation of the longitudinal coat does not occur until "rotation" is complete.)

The liver, growing within the ventral mesogastrium, becomes a largely right-sided abdominal organ; the spleen, appearing within the dorsal mesogastrium, lies on the left (Fig. 11-4).

MIDGUT AND DORSAL MESENTERY

At the time of appearance of the omental bursa, the vitelline duct is undergoing a rapid reduction in size. The attachment of the vitelline duct to the gut keeps the middle part of the intestinal tract close to the umbilicus (Fig. 11-2). The resultant U-shaped segment of intestine is the *midgut loop*. It is linked to the stomach by the narrow *duodenum*.

During the sixth week of gestation the midgut begins to lengthen prodigiously. At this time the liver is also growing at an enormous rate; it fills the greater part of the abdominal cavity. Accommodation for the gut must be sought elsewhere, and it is found *within the umbilical cord*. The lengthening intestine is extruded into a loculus of embryonic coelom within the cord, constituting the remarkable "physiologic hernia of the midgut" (Fig. 11-8).

As first the midgut forms a simple loop within the umbilical cord, having cranial and caudal limbs. The caudal limb is identified by a swelling—the primitive *cecum*—on its outer (antimesenteric) aspect.

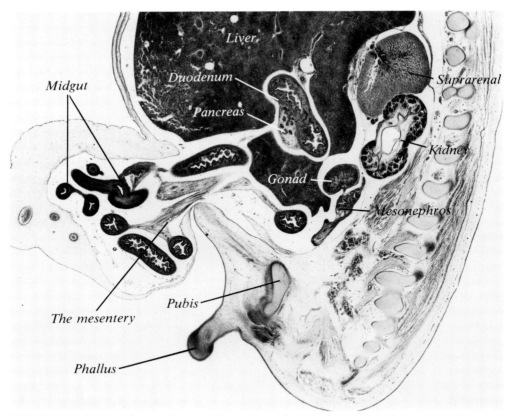

FIG. 11-8. Sagittal section at nine weeks' gestation, showing the physiologic hernia of the midgut. (Carnegie Collection) (x20)

FIG. 11-9. Rotation of the midgut loop.
A. The arrangement immediately following return to the abdominal cavity.
B. The adult arrangement; stippled areas denote fusion of the mesentery with the posterior abdominal wall. The greater omentum is unduly short; it normally grows down to overlie the transverse colon and small intestine.

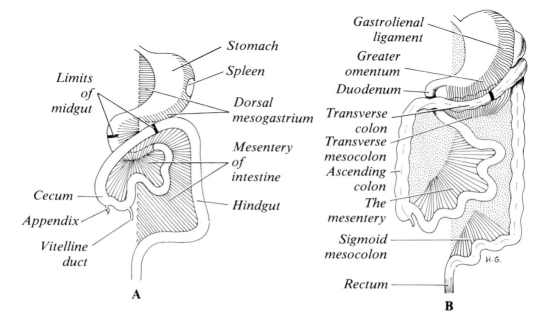

ROTATION OF THE GUT

Even as it enters the umbilical cord, the midgut loop begins to twist on itself. The axis of rotation is that of the superior mesenteric artery, which runs from the aorta to the apex of the loop (Fig. 11-2). When observed from in front, the direction of rotation is counter-clockwise. A rotation of 180 degrees carries the caudal limb to the left of the cranial limb, and then above it. The cecal region rotates through a further 90 degrees, coming to lie on the right-hand side (Fig 11-9A). At the same time the (original) cranial limb is elongating rapidly to form the coiled *jejunum* and *ileum*.

By the 10th to 12th week the capacity of the abdomen has increased by a reduction in the rate of growth of the liver. The intestine slides back into the peritoneal cavity. The manner of return of the midgut is not random, but follows a well-ordered pattern. The small intestine returns first and occupies the central abdomen; the hindgut, displaced towards the left by the small intestine, forms the descending and sigmoid portions of the colon. The cecum is the widest section of the gut and it is held within the extraembryonic loculus until last. It retains its rotated condition, however, coming to occupy the right side of the abdomen directly below the liver. At this time the right lobe of the liver extends to the lower lumbar level, and the cecum lies in its rightful place. The segment comprising both the ascending and the transverse elements of the colon extends obliquely to the left, being anchored to the second stage of the duodenum. This arrangement is usually still present at birth. The definitive ascending colon makes its appearance as the duodenum and cecum retreat from one another while the posterior abdominal wall elongates progressively (Fig. 11-9B).

THE APPENDIX

The primitive cecum elongates into tubular form (Fig. 11-10). Its distal part lags behind the rest, creating the *vermiform appendix*. Its proximal part develops three teniae of longitudinal muscle continuous with those of the colon. The teniae converge on the apex of the cone-shaped cecum and they invest the appendix. The further growth of the cecum is asymmetrical. Its medial wall adheres for a time to the surface of the ileum, and grows slowly. Its lateral wall bulges outwards progressively. The lateral expansion continues for several years after birth, the appendix being displaced to the medial side of the cecum. However, the three teniae, converging upon the root of the appendix, continue to indicate the original apex of the cecum.

FATE OF THE DORSAL MESENTERY

The attachment of the dorsal mesentery to the posterior abdominal wall is greatly modified following the return of the midgut loop. Figure 11-11 illustrates the stages of the dorsal mesentery's history.

FIG. 11-10. The vermiform appendix: **A**, at 10 weeks; **B**, at birth; **C**, adult.

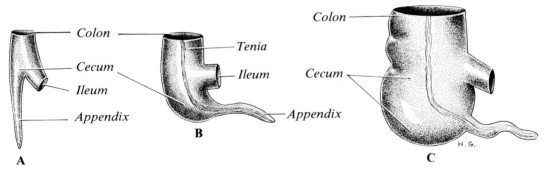

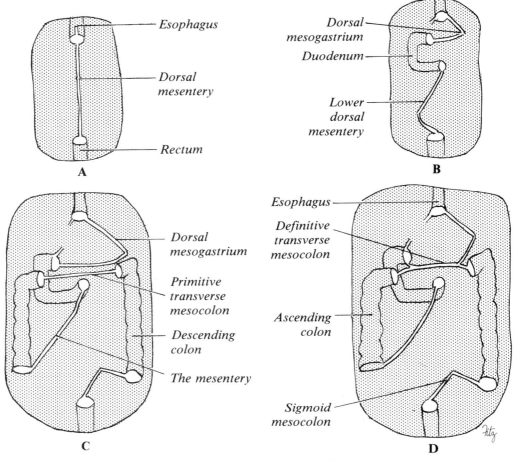

FIG. 11-11. The posterior abdominal wall, showing transformation of the dorsal mesentery of the gastrointestinal tract.

FIG. 11-12. Sagittal sections to show transformation of the dorsal mesogastrium: **A,** before fusion; **B,** after fusion with primitive transverse mesocolon.

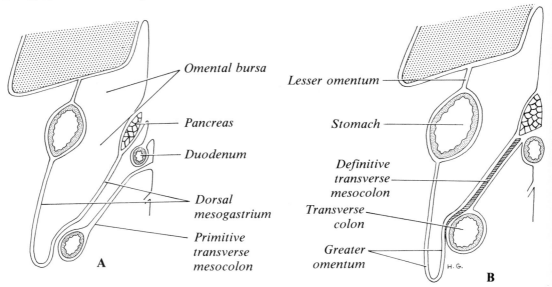

A. At first the dorsal mesentery occupies the sagittal plane.

B. The colon presses the duodenum against the posterior abdominal wall. The duodenal mesentery is absorbed and this segment of the gut becomes retroperitoneal. The dorsal mesentery then has two parts—the dorsal mesogastrium (which has become V-shaped) extending from the esophagus to the upper end of the duodenum, and the *lower dorsal mesentery* which connects the lower end of the duodenum to the rectum, and suspends the jejunum, ileum, and colon.

C. The descending colon loses its mesentery and becomes retroperitoneal. The ascending colon (as this forms) also becomes retroperitoneal. The lower dorsal mesentery then has three parts: (**a**) *the mesentery of the small intestine;* (**b**) *the primitive transverse mesocolon;* and (**c**) *the sigmoid mesocolon.*

D. The transverse mesocolon is parallel to the lower, horizontal part of the dorsal mesogastrium. The two peritoneal folds come together to form the *definitive transverse mesocolon* (Fig. 11-12). The fusion accounts for the bifurcation observed at the left and right ends of the attachment of the mesocolon in the adult.

DORSAL MESOGASTRIUM AND SPLEEN

Duodenal fixation confers the characteristic V shape upon the dorsal mesogastrium. The mesogastrium then has left and inferior parts attached to the corresponding parts of the greater curvature of the stomach.

The left part is transformed by the growth of the spleen and left kidney. The spleen arises in the sixth week of gestation as an aggregation of reticular mesenchymal cells within the left part of the dorsal mesogastrium (Fig. 11-2). In later pregnancy the splenic reticulum is infiltrated by lymphocytes that multiply to form the lymph follicles. The expanding spleen bulges to the left, projecting into the greater peritoneal sac. The hilus of the spleen marks the left boundary of the omental bursa. The developing left kidney abuts against the mesogastrium and causes the greater sac to be obliterated in this region. The left part of the dorsal mesogastrium then comprises the *gastrolienal ligament,* passing from stomach to spleen, and the *lienorenal ligament,* passing from spleen to kidney.

The inferior part of the dorsal mesogastrium is folded on itself where it hangs down ventral to the transverse colon (Fig. 11-12). It adheres to the transverse colon and mesocolon so that these become part of the posterior wall of the lesser sac. After birth, the mesogastrium hangs a progressively greater distance below the transverse colon, forming the *greater omentum.* Its small size in the child is clinically significant, because it is unable as yet to reach the appendix to seal off a threatened perforation in the course of acute appendicitis.

PORTAL VEIN

The portal venous system drains the entire alimentary tract below the diaphragm. The portal vein is formed by segments of the left and right vitelline veins, which anastomose below, within, and above the duodenum in the form of a figure eight (Fig. 11-13A). As the third (horizontal) stage of the duodenum becomes fixed to the posterior abdominal wall, the dorsal venous loop is lost here. Above, it is the ventral loop that is lost. The splenic vein joints the middle anastomosis (Fig. 11-13B).

PANCREAS

The *ventral* pancreas arises from the hepatic diverticulum as a solid bud of endodermal cells. The *dorsal* pancreas arises directly from the duodenal endoderm (Fig. 11-13A) and burrows into the dorsal mesogastrium.

Unequal growth of the duodenal wall carries the bile duct, and with it the ventral pancreas, first to its dorsal and later to its left aspect (Fig. 11-13B). Paradoxically, the ventral pancreas is then dorsal, and lies behind the superior mesenteric vein. The larger dorsal pancreas is in front of the splenic and portal veins. The ventral outgrowth forms the lower part of the head of the pancreas, including the *uncinate process*. The dorsal one forms the remainder of the gland.

The pancreas is carried to the posterior abdominal wall together with the splenic vessels, and adheres to it.

Since the *main pancreatic duct* of the adult enters the gut in common with the bile duct, and since the bulk of the gland arises directly from the duodenum, it follows that the duct system must be radically changed during development. The change is the result of take-over of the smaller drainage system by the larger one. The terminal part of the dorsal pancreatic duct usually persists as the small *accessory pancreatic duct* (Fig. 11-13C).

SMALL INTESTINE

The intense mitotic activity of the duodenal epithelium, in producing the hepatic and dorsal pancreatic diverticula, interrupts the lumen at this level during the fifth and sixth weeks of

FIG. 11-13. Portal vein, biliary tract, and pancreas.

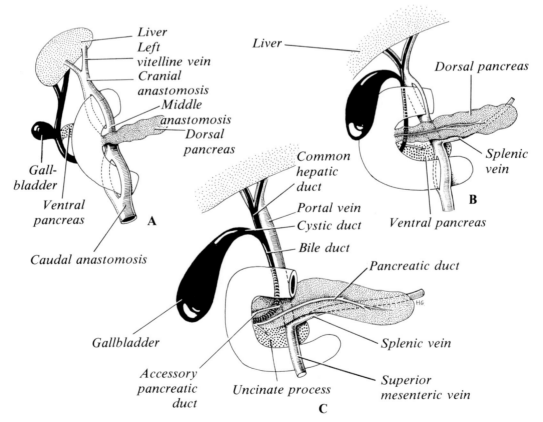

gestation. These outgrowths terminate for a time in blind endodermal pockets within the duodenum. Duodenal development is further complicated by a wave of growth and differentiation that sweeps along its entire length, narrowing and often duplicating its lumen. By the end of the seventh week the definitive lumen has been established by the coalescence of intercellular spaces in the endodermal core, the spaces being created by localized cellular death.

The lumen of the ileum is also normally occluded during the extremely rapid elongation of the ileum within the umbilical cord.

INTERMEDIATE MESODERM

The intermediate mesoderm is the cell column that links the paraxial mesoderm to the lateral plate. At first it shows no evidence of segmentation, detaching itself from the somites as these appear. During lateral flexion it separates also from the lateral plate, coming to lie on either side of the root of the dorsal mesentery (Fig. 11-1). Here it gives rise to 1) the cortex of the suprarenal glands, 2) the kidneys, 3) the gonads, and 4) the genital ducts.

SUPRARENAL GLANDS

The suprarenal glands have a dual origin. The *cortex* develops from the intermediate mesoderm. The medulla is ectodermal, arising directly from the neural crest.

During the sixth week the surface epithelium of the intermediate mesoderm, beside the root of the dorsal mesentery, forms the rudiment of the suprarenal cortex. The rudiment gives rise to an outer rim of cells—the precursor of the adult cortex—and an inner, "fetal" cortex which persists throughout fetal life and which undergoes a sudden, unexplained degeneration at or shortly after full term. The function of the "fetal" cortex is unknown. It is absent in anencephaly (Chapter 12), in which the hypothalamic–pituitary pathway is defective.

The adult cortical rim differentiates into *zona glomerulosa* and *zona fascicularis* by the 12th week, at which time it appears to produce its full range of steroid hormones. The *zona reticularis* is derived later from the zona fasciculata.

The suprarenal medulla is composed of *chromaffin cells,* so called because of their affinity for chrome salts. They secrete epinephrine and norepinephrine, reflecting their origin from neurons of the sympathetic nervous system. The medulla makes its appearance during the seventh week, when neuroblasts migrate from the lower thoracic and upper lumbar sympathetic ganglia into the interior of the cortical primordium. They become scattered throughout the cortex until the fetal element degenerates; then they accumulate around the central vein and establish the definitive medulla. Preganglionic nerve fibers travel in the splanchnic nerves and synapse directly upon them.

GENITOURINARY SYSTEM

The development of the genitourinary system is complex. The following features should be borne in mind while reading the chronological account which follows:

1. Three successive renal systems—the first two vestigial—appear in man. They are the *pronephros,* the *mesonephros,* and the *metanephros* or permanent kidney.
2. The gonad are homologous, the earliest stages of testicular and ovarian development being indistinguishable.
3. The genital ducts are *not* homologous. The male duct is the *mesonephric (wolffian) duct* —surprisingly, a derivative of the renal excretory system. That of the female is the

paramesonephric (*müllerian*) *duct.* However, both ducts make an appearance in both sexes; the "inappropriate" duct later degenerates almost entirely.

4. The *ureters* are a third pair of ducts that arise as sprouts from the mesonephric ducts.

PRONEPHROS

During the early somite period the cells of the intermediate mesoderm in the cervical region group themselves around a central *pronephric duct,* which quickly extends through the thoracic and abdominal intermediate mesoderm to open into the side wall of the cloaca. In larval amphibia and in some fishes the pronephros is the definitive kidney, composed of segmentally arranged tubules passing from the coelomic cavity to the pronephric duct. In man the pronephros is vestigial, comprising scattered cell cords in the cervical region. These cords acquire no lumen, nor do they make contact with their duct. By the end of the somite period (30 days) they have disappeared, together with the cervical part of the pronephric duct.

MESONEPHROS

The mesonephros makes its appearance as the pronephros wanes. It is the definitive kidney of amphibia and of most fishes. It consists of renal tubules formed by the intermediate mesoderm in the thoracolumbar region. Their proximal (medial) ends are invaginated by capillary tufts developing *in situ,* and these are fed by branches of some 20 arteries from each side of the aorta. Their distal ends open into the pronephric duct, which is then known as the *mesonephric duct* (Fig. 11-14).

THE KIDNEY (METANEPHROS)

The ureteric bud arises from the dorsal aspect of the mesonephric duct, close to the point of entry of the duct into the cloaca. The bud extends into the intermediate mesoderm behind

FIG. 11-14. The mesonephros early in the sixth week of gestation. (Cambridge Collection) (x150)

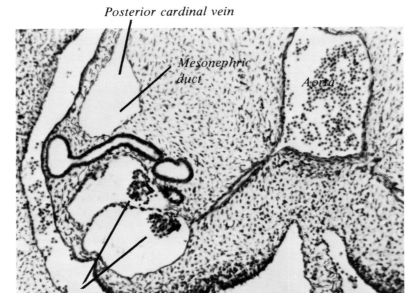

the lower end of the mesonephros. Its stalk acquires a lumen to become the *ureter* proper. The lumen invades the advancing ureteric bud and dilates to form the *renal pelvis*. The adjacent cells of the intermediate mesoderm multiply to form the *metanephric cap*, which invests the renal pelvis (Figs. 11-15 and 11-16).

The ureteric bud divides dichotomously to form successive generations of collecting tubules. The first three to four tubular generations enlarge and become confluent to form the *major calyces*. The second four generations coalesce to form the *minor calyces*. The minor calyces expand in cuplike fashion, each receiving some sixteen tubules of the ninth order. The tubules of the ninth to sixteenth order remain separate to form the definitive *collecting tubules* of the kidney. The metanephric cap arranges itself in lobules in relation to the minor calyces. Lobulation diminishes with continued differentiation, but it is still recognizable in the kidney of the newborn.

A cluster of metanephric cells forms at the tip of each collecting duct. This differentiates into a *nephron,* comprising Bowman's capsule, proximal convoluted tubule, loop of Henle, and distal convoluted tubule. Bowman's capsule is invaginated by a capillary tuft to complete the renal corpuscle. Each distal convoluted tubule opens into an adjacent collecting tubule.

If the metanephric primordium is grown in tissue culture, the epithelial component proceeds to form collecting tubules and the investing mesenchyme to form recognizable nephrons. However, if the two elements are separated by tryptic digestion, organogenesis fails altogether. It appears that branching of the ureteric bud is dependent upon induction by the metanephric cap, and that development of nephrons depends in turn upon induction by the collecting tubules.

Ascent of the Kidneys

At first the kidneys lie in front of the sacrum, and the renal corpuscles are fed by the internal iliac artery. The intermediate mesoderm contributes to the metanephric cap from above, so that renal enlargement occurs in a cranial direction (Fig. 11-17). The kidneys attain their adult position during the eighth week. As they ascend, they are supplied successively by

FIG. 11-15. The kidneys at 10 weeks. (Cambridge Collection) (x15)

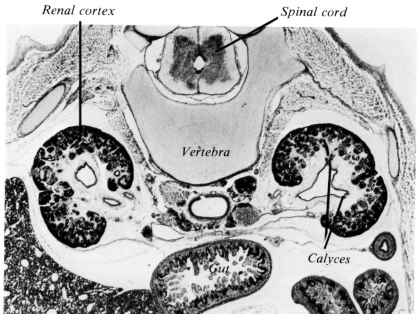

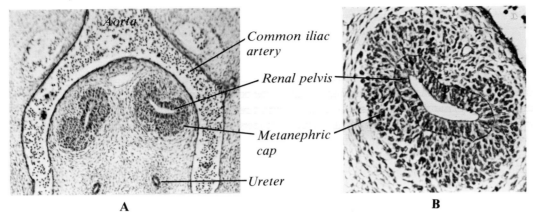

FIG. 11-16. The metanephros at the pelvic brim at six weeks (Cambridge Collection) (**A**, x100; **B**, x250)

FIG. 11-17. Ascent of the kidneys: **A**, sixth week; **B**, seven weeks; **C**, eight weeks. (Adapted from Kelly HA and Burnam CF: in Diseases of the Kidneys, Ureters and Bladder, Vol. 1. New York, Appleton, Century Crofts, 1922, p 180)

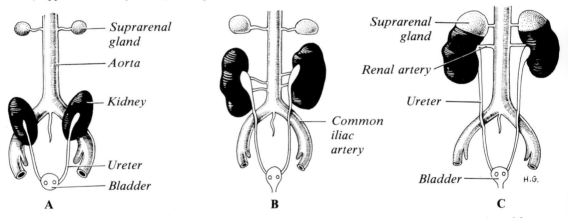

twigs from the common iliac artery and lower abdominal aorta. These twigs are replaced by the definitive *renal arteries*. The kidneys also rotate during ascent, the renal pelvis changing from an anterior to a medial position (Fig. 11-17).

The metanephros functions from midgestation onwards. The urine is excreted into the amniotic cavity and much of it is transferred across the amnion to the placenta. Some is swallowed by the fetus, absorbed from the fetal alimentary tract, and its waste products taken to the placenta through the fetal circulation. The main function of the kidneys *in utero* appears to be the production of the protective cushion of amniotic fluid. In *bilateral renal agenesis* (a very rare condition in which the kidneys do not develop), little or no amniotic fluid is present at full term. However, fetal electrolytic stability is not impaired, being controlled by placental exchange. Infants thus afflicted survive only a few days after birth.

EARLY STAGES OF TESTICULAR AND OVARIAN DEVELOPMENT

Gonads

It is now accepted that the germ cells do not arise in the gonad itself, but migrate there from the yolk sac. In early somite embryos about 100 germ cells are found among the endodermal cells of the yolk sac, close to the allantois (Fig. 11-18). These cells become ameboid and, dividing as they go, travel by the dorsal mesentery to the intermediate mesoderm, there to await the development of the gonad. Therefore, the germ cells arise either from the yolk sac endoderm or from stem cells that become lodged there. It is clear that *one of the first duties of the differentiating blastocyst is to set aside the cells that will give rise to the next human generation.*

During the fifth week the coelomic surface epithelium of the intermediate mesoderm thickens to become the *germinal epithelium,* so styled when it was thought to give rise to the germ cells. From the epithelium, strands of cells—the *sex cords*—grow into the underlying mesoderm. Germ cells migrate along the cords and come to occupy both the outer (cortical) and inner (medullary) part of the gonad.

Until the seventh week the gonads are "different," (Fig. 11-23A) *i.e.,* they are not recognizably male or female, although the sex of the embryo can, of course, be determined from the 18th day after fertilization onwards by observation of the sex chromatin. The female gonad remains "indifferent" until mid-gestation, whereas the male one differentiates rapidly.

Testis. During the seventh and eighth weeks of gestation the cortical germ cells and sex cords of male embryos degenerate. In the medulla the sex cords become prominent, forming the primitive *seminiferous tubules* (Fig. 11-19). The tubules comprise strands of interstitial cells (of Leydig) and primordial male germ cells (spermatogonia). The spermatogonia lie dormant until the tenth postnatal year, at which time the tubules acquire a lumen and the germ cells initiate spermatogenesis.

The androgen-secreting interstitial cells increase in number until the 24th week, after which their numbers are greatly reduced. Their function will be considered with the development of the genital duct system (genital tract).

The Urogenital Union. About a dozen tubules of the mesonephros are preserved in the male. Their glomeruli are shed, and their proximal ends join the tubules of the testis. These mesonephric tubules become the *efferent ductules* of the testis. The mesonephric duct, into which the ductules empty, is now the *ductus deferens* (Fig. 11-23B). The proximal part of the mesonephric duct becomes highly convoluted to form the *epididymis.* Near its entry into the urethra, the distal end is incorporated into the developing prostate as the *ejaculatory*

FIG. 11-18. Transverse section early in the fifth week of gestation showing migrating germ cells. (From Witschi E: Contrib Embryol Carnegie Inst 32:67–80, 1948, by courtesy of the Carnegie Institution) (x75)

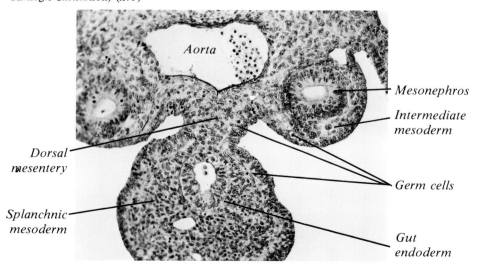

Aorta

Mesonephros

Intermediate mesoderm

Germ cells

Dorsal mesentery

Splanchnic mesoderm

Gut endoderm

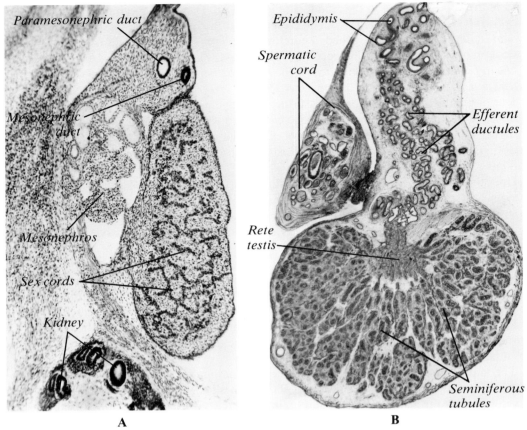

FIG. 11-19. Transverse section of testis and adjacent structures: **A**, at eight weeks; **B**, at 20 weeks. (University of Washington Collection) (**A**, x70; **B**, x50)

duct. Directly behind the prostate a diverticulum from the duct gives rise to the *seminal vesicle.*

In the female the mesonephric ducts regress, perhaps under the influence of circulating estrogen. Tiny remnants of mesonephric tissue may persist beside the ovary as the *epoophoron,* and in the vaginal wall as a Gärtner's cyst (Fig. 11-23C).

Ovary. The pattern here is the reverse of testicular development—the cortex grows, while the medulla undergoes regression.

The female primordial germ cells are the oogonia. The signal for ovarian differentiation is the enlargement of thousands of oogonia, under the influence of placental gonadotropic hormone. The enlarged oogonia as called *primary oocytes,* and the sex cords invest each one with follicular epithelium (Fig. 11-20). The interstitial mesenchyme forms the ovarian stroma.

A few sex cords, with Leydig cells, normally persist in the ovarian medulla until shortly before birth. Certain virilizing tumors of adult females are thought to arise from persistent Leydig cells.

SUBDIVISION OF THE CLOACA

The cloaca is the common endodermal chamber into which the hindgut and allantois open. Outside the cloacal membrane lies an ectodermal depression called the *proctodeum* (Fig. 11-22A), which is comparable to the stomodeum at the other extremity of the gut.

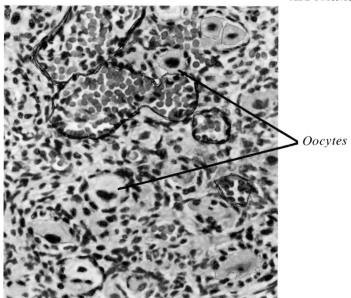

Oocytes

FIG. 11-20. Ovarian cortex of a two-year-old girl. (Section kindly supplied by Dr Carl Mottet) (x300)

The caudal mesoderm has been seen to extend rostrally on each side of the allantois to enter the lower abdominal wall, early in the fourth week (Fig. 6-15). During the fifth week the mesoderm accumulates on the dorsal side of the allantois as the *urorectal septum* (Fig. 11-22B). The septum grows caudally to meet the cloacal membrane, splitting the cloaca into the *urogenital sinus* ventrally, and the *rectum* dorsally. The corresponding parts of the divided cloacal membrane are the *urogenital membrane* and the *anal membrane*. The mesonephric duct opens into the urogenital sinus.

The pelvic extensions of the coelom establish the pelvic portion of the peritoneal cavity.

THE PARAMESONEPHRIC DUCTS

Shortly before the gonad undergoes sexual dimorphism, the coelomic epithelium lateral to the cephalic extremity of the mesonephric duct shows a funnel-shaped invagination; this is the primordium of the *paramesonephric (müllerian) duct*. The mouth of the funnel is the ostium (fimbriated end) of the uterine tube. Its blind end burrows in a caudal direction, becoming canalized from above as it does so (Fig. 11-21).

At the lower pole of the mesonephros the paramesonephric ducts pass ventral to the mesonephric ducts and come together. They fuse between rectum and urogenital sinus. The *uterine canal,* formed by the fused ducts, abuts blindly on the dorsal wall of the urogenital sinus. Each paramesonephric duct is suspended from the mesonephros by a short mesentery, and the medial swing of the two mesenteries creates a complete transverse partition—the *urogenital septum*—between urogenital sinus and rectum. The urogenital septum in the female is the precursor of the *broad ligaments of the uterus* (Fig. 11-23C).

The paramesonephric ducts display upper vertical, intermediate horizontal, and lower (conjoined) vertical segments (Fig. 11-23). In females, the upper segments form the epithelium of the uterine tubes; the intermediate and lower segments form the epithelium of the body and cervix of the uterus. The cavity of the uterus is bicornuate, *i.e.,* Y-shaped, until the third month; later, the fundus arises as an upward expansion.

In males, the cranial end of a paramesonephric duct may form the insignificant *appendix testis,* and the caudal end of the uterine canal helps to form the *prostatic utricle* (Fig. 11-23B).

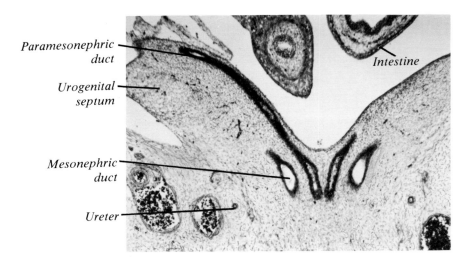

Paramesonephric duct

Intestine

Urogenital septum

Mesonephric duct

Ureter

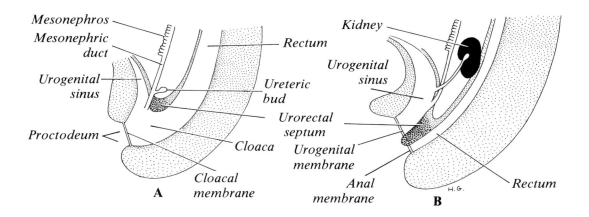

Mesonephros

Mesonephric duct

Kidney

Rectum

Urogenital sinus

Urogenital sinus

Ureteric bud

Proctodeum

Urorectal septum

Cloaca

Urogenital membrane

Cloacal membrane

Anal membrane

Rectum

A

B

BLADDER AND URETHRA

The urogenital sinus shows an expansion, the *primitive bladder,* above the level of the mesonephric ducts. The allantois, linking the apex of the bladder to the umbilicus, undergoes early regression; its lumen disappears, the surrounding mesoderm persisting as the fibrous *urachus.*

The primitive bladder gradually incorporates the lower ends of the mesonephric ducts, and the ureters then open directly into it. The *definitive bladder* is established by the differentiation of its smooth muscle wall from the surrounding mesoderm. The openings of the mesonephric ducts are carried caudally to the urethra (Fig. 11-22B). As they migrate the ducts contribute mesodermal epithelium to the base of the bladder and to the posterior wall of the urethra; this epithelium is finally replaced by bladder endoderm.

The caudal mesoderm, having contributed to the lower abdominal wall and to the urorectal septum, enlarges *in situ* to form the *genital tubercle.* The genital tubercle extends ventrally as the *phallus,* and the urogenital sinus is continued forwards below it. The urogenital sinus below the bladder then has two parts—a narrow, vertical *pelvic part* behind the phallus, and a horizontal *phallic part* below it (Fig. 11-24). The phallic part is slot-shaped in the sagittal plane; it is floored by the urogenital membrane (Figs. 11-24A and 11-25A). In the seventh week the membrane disintegrates and the phallic part of the sinus is thrown open (Figs. 11-24B and 11-25B).

From the pelvic part of the sinus, epithelial buds penetrate the surrounding mesoderm. In the female they give rise to the paraurethral glands. In the male the outgrowths proliferate further to form the glandular tissue of the *prostate*. The prostate is completed by a fibro-muscular contribution from the mesoderm. The glands of the median lobe of the prostate are derived from the posterior urethral wall; these may well be of mesodermal origin, from mesonephric duct epithelium. The response of the adult median lobe to hormonal stimulation, especially by estrogens, differs from that of the remainder of the prostate. This feature may in some way be related to an origin from a different germ layer.

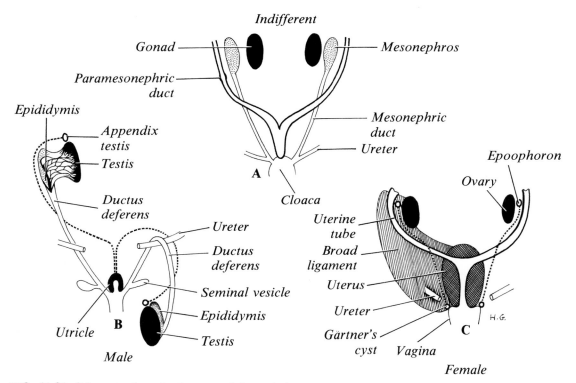

FIG. 11-23. Scheme to show development of the genital tracts.

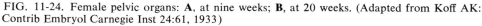

FIG. 11-24. Female pelvic organs: **A**, at nine weeks; **B**, at 20 weeks. (Adapted from Koff AK: Contrib Embryol Carnegie Inst 24:61, 1933)

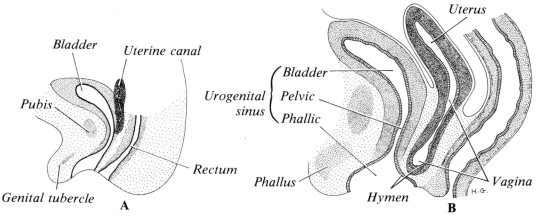

EXTERNAL GENITALIA

Examination of the perineum late in the third month shows no evidence of sexual divergence. The phallic urethra is an open endodermal trough, flanked by the *urogenital folds* derived from the adjacent mesenchyme. More laterally, the mesenchyme forms *labioscrotal folds* as well. From the anterior (distal) extremity of the phallic part of the urogenital sinus a keel-shaped growth of endodermal cells—the *urethral plate*—penetrates the genital tubercle (Fig. 11-25). The urogenital folds are carried along the under surface of the lengthening phallus to make a trough, the *urogenital groove,* which is lined centrally by the urethral plate.

The fate of the urogenital and labioscrotal folds is quite different in the two sexes. In the male, under androgenic hormonal stimulation, the matching pairs come together in the midline, but in the female they stay apart.

MALE EXTERNAL GENITALIA

The male phallus elongates progressively to form the *penis*. The urogenital folds are carried along its under surface. The urethral plate disintegrates, deepening the urogenital groove (Fig. 11-26A). The urogenital folds meet below the groove to form the *spongy urethra*. Behind, they meet below the phallic part of the urogenital sinus to complete the *urethral bulb.*

At first, the urethra opens behind the terminal expansion of the penis called the *glans*. During the fourth month an ectodermal invagination from the tip of the glans grows in to join the spongy urethra, forming most of the *glandular urethra*. The urogenital groove closes completely, and the urethral canal is carried forwards to the tip of the penis (Fig. 11-26B).

The *prepuce* (foreskin) develops as a collarlike outgrowth of skin from the base of the glans.

The *labioscrotal folds* form the *scrotum* on each side. They enlarge and come together below the bulb of the urethra. The line of fusion of the paired urogenital folds, and of the paired labioscrotal folds, is marked by the *anogenital raphe* in the midline (Fig. 11-26B).

FEMALE EXTERNAL GENITALIA

The female external genitalia arise by the growth *in situ* of the urogenital and labioscrotal folds (Fig. 11-27A). The phallus swells to form the *clitoris*. The small urethral plate breaks

FIG. 11-25. External genitalia, indifferent stages. In **B** the urogenital and anal membranes have broken down.

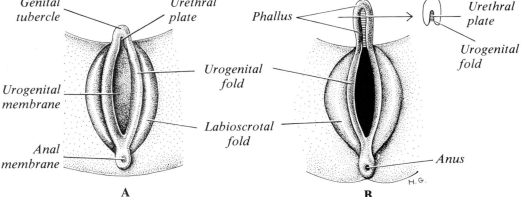

| A | B |

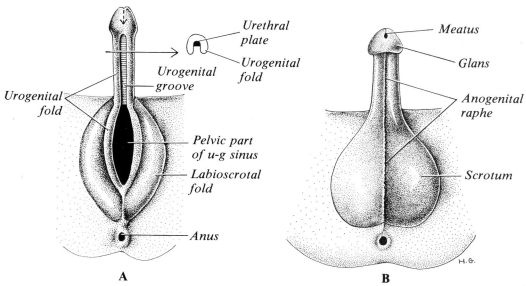

FIG. 11-26. Male external genitalia.
A. The **arrow** in the glans penis indicates ingrowth of ectoderm to form the glandular urethra.
B. Following the union of urogenital and labioscrotal folds.

FIG. 11-27. Formation of female external genitalia.

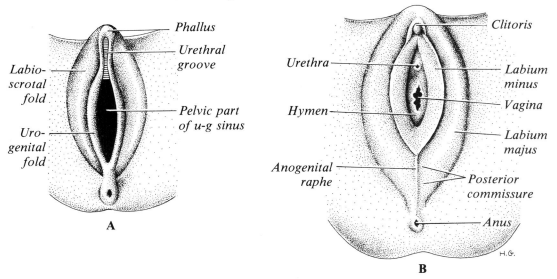

down. The phallic part of the urogenital sinus, and the urogenital groove, remain open as the *vestibule*. The urogenital folds flank the vestibule as the *labia minora*. The labioscrotal folds form the *labia majora*. These folds do come together between anus and vestibule to establish the *posterior commissure* (Fig. 11-27B).

VAGINA

The *vaginal plate* is a dense column of cells formed in the female at the junction of the uterine canal with the urogenital sinus. The plate lengthens in both cranial and caudal directions. In growing cranially, it pushes the uterus ahead of it, so that the body of the uterus comes to lie on the upper surface of the bladder. In growing caudally, it migrates down the posterior wall of the urogenital sinus (Fig. 11-24).

Studies on lower mammals suggest that the upper three-fifths of the vaginal plate are derived from paramesonephric epithelium, and the lower two-fifths from urogenital sinus epithelium.

The vaginal lumen is formed by the canalization of the vaginal plate from the vestibule upwards. The lumen extends around the cervix uteri to define the *vaginal fornices*. The *hymen* is the partition between the vagina and the vestibule (Fig. 11-24B). It breaks down in the perinatal period.

LATER DEVELOPMENT OF GENITAL TRACT

THE GUBERNACULUM

The mesentery of the paramesonephric duct becomes attached to the lower abdominal wall by the *inguinal fold* of mesoderm. A fibrous cord, the *gubernaculum,* develops within the fold. The ventral end of the gubernaculum reaches the inguinal region and the dorsal end gains attachment to the gonad (Fig. 11-28). The gubernaculum undergoes little increase in length, and it anchors the gonad while the trunk continues to grow. By the seventh month the relative descent of the gonad has brought it to the corresponding iliac fossa. The gubernaculum undergoes a gelatinous enlargement, maintaining a defect—the *inguinal canal*—in the abdominal wall. A peritoneal diverticulum, the *processus vaginalis,* grows alongside the gubernaculum to reach the scrotum or labium majus (Fig. 11-29A).

FIG. 11-28. **A.** Male genitourinary system at 12 weeks.
B. Female genitourinary system at 12 weeks. (From dissections)

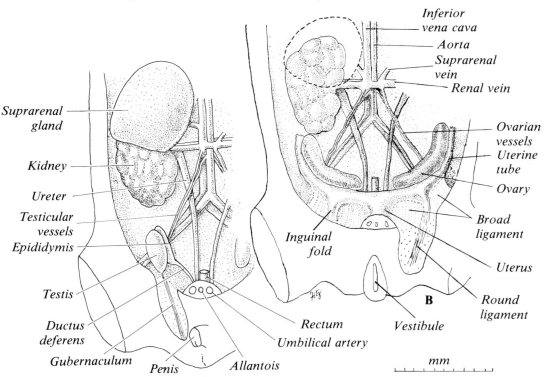

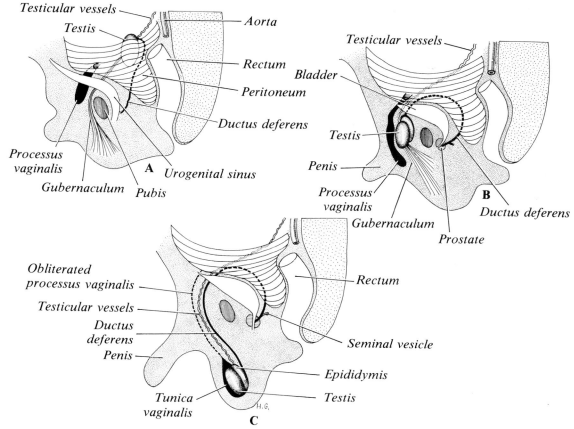

FIG. 11-29. Descent of testis and formation of the spermatic cord. (Adapted in part from Tuchmann-Duplessis H, Haegel P: Illustrated Human Embryology, Vol. 2, Paris, Masson et Cie, 1972, p 87)

TESTIS

During the final two months of gestation the testis descends along the inguinal canal, behind the processus vaginalis (Fig. 11-29B). Descent to the scrotum is usually completed before term; however, it may lie anywhere along the inguinal canal at birth, gaining the scrotum during the first postnatal year. The ductus deferens and the testicular vessels, nerves, and lymphatics accompany the testis; collectively, they constitute the *spermatic cord*. The processus vaginalis is normally obliterated along the inguinal canal when the testis has passed through. Its blind extremity forms the *tunica vaginalis* of the testis (Fig. 11-29C).

OVARY

The gubernaculum of the ovary gains a secondary, permanent attachment to the tubouterine junction. Thus anchored, the gubernaculum of the female does not shorten, but persists as the *round ligament of the uterus*. Its ovarian attachment forms the *ligament of the ovary*.

CONTROL OF SEX DIFFERENTIATION

Whatever the genetic sex of the individual, the reproductive system passes through an indifferent, ambisexual phase before becoming recognizably male or female. The Y chromosome is evidently responsible for intiating morphogenesis of the testis, because normal testicular development ocurs only in its presence. Individuals with abnormal chromosome complements (such as XXY or XXXY), but carrying a Y chromosome, usually form a male genital system.

The testis or ovary, once formed, directs the further development of the genital tract. Testicular androgens promote the continued growth of the mesonephric ducts and the masculinization of the external genitalia; and they suppress the paramesonephric ducts (Fig. 11-30). The androgens are secreted by the interstitial cells of the testis, which reach their maximal development during this critical period. Early removal of the testis, *i.e.,* castration, in experimental animals is followed by loss of the mesonephric ducts and the development of a female-type genital tract and external genitalia. It is of interest here that *female* fetuses with precocious development of the suprarenal cortex (adrenal cortical hyperplasia) may exhibit a masculinization of the external genitalia at birth. This result is probably due to production of suprarenal androgens in excessive amounts.

Ovarian estrogens promote the growth of the female genital tract. An ovariectomized female embryo will form a female genital tract of less than normal size.

RECTUM AND ANAL CANAL

The rectum, cut off from the urogenital sinus by the urorectal system, adapts its shape to the curvature of the developing sacrum. Its lining epithelium and glands are derived from cloacal endoderm. The surrounding mesoderm forms the circular and longitudinal muscle coats (Fig. 11-31), and the ganglia of Auerbach's plexus invade it from the neural crest.

The anal membrane lies at the bottom of the *anal pit,* an ectoderm-lined depression created by a dorsal extension of the urogenital fold (Fig. 11-25). During the seventh week the membrane breaks down and the rectum opens into the amniotic sac. The *pectinate line,* at the middle of the anal canal, probably represents the former site of attachment of the anal membrane; below this level the epithelium is stratified and is innervated by somatic nerve fibers. Above it, the epithelium is columnar and is supplied by visceral afferent fibers traveling in the autonomic nervous system.

INFERIOR VENA CAVA

The development of the inferior vena cava is complex. In addition to the posterior cardinal veins, as many as five paired longitudinal channels develop on the posterior abdominal wall; these anastomose freely with one another. The fate of all these channels is still in dispute, but it is clear at least that the construction of the inferior vena cava entails the replacement

FIG. 11-30. Control of sex differentiation.

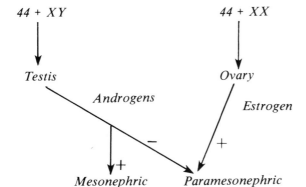

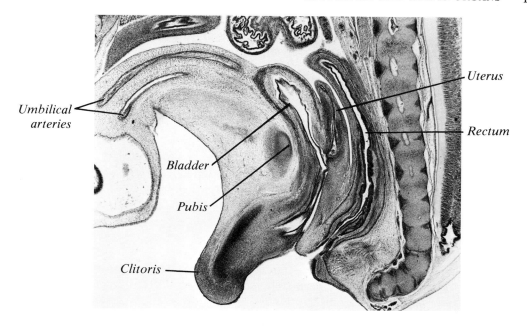

Umbilical
arteries

Uterus

Rectum

Bladder

Pubis

Clitoris

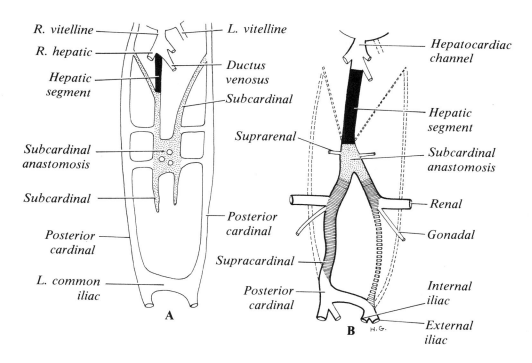

R. vitelline

R. hepatic

Hepatic
segment

Subcardinal
anastomosis

Subcardinal

Posterior
cardinal

L. common
iliac

L. vitelline

Ductus
venosus

Subcardinal

Posterior
cardinal

A

Hepatocardiac
channel

Hepatic
segment

Subcardinal
anastomosis

Renal

Gonadal

Suprarenal

Supracardinal

Posterior
cardinal

Internal
iliac

External
iliac

B   H.G.

of the posterior cardinal system by two new veins—the *right subcardinal* and the *right supracardinal* (Fig. 11-32A).

The subcardinal veins appear on the medial side of the mesonephroi and anastomose freely with the posterior cardinals. The right subcardinal sends a vascular bud—the *hepatic segment*—to join the hepatocardiac channel. The subcardinals anastomose in front of the abdominal aorta. The supracardinal veins appear between the posterior cardinal and the subcardinal, and they are linked to both. The veins of the permanent kidneys and gonads enter the supracardinals.

The component parts of the inferior vena cava, from above downward, are, therefore, as follows: 1) the hepatocardiac channel; 2) the hepatic segment; 3) the subcardinal anastomotic segment; 4) the supracardinal segment; and 5) the posterior cardinal segment (Fig. 11-32B).

ABNORMALITIES

LIVER AND GALLBLADDER

Anomalies of the cystic and hepatic ducts are commonplace and are derived from the variable mode of branching of the original hepatic diverticulum. Rarely, the cystic branch of the diverticulum may fail altogether, leading to *absence of the gallbladder.* The hepatic diverticulum or its branches may fail to acquire a lumen, causing *atresia* of the biliary or cystic ducts. Atresia of the common bile duct leads to jaundice which appears shortly after birth and becomes progressively deeper.

Should the lumen of the duodenum or ileum fail to reappear towards the end of the second month, *congenital atresia* will result, with complete intestinal obstruction. Partial failure will produce *intestinal stenosis.* The point of entry of the bile duct is the most common site of atresia.

Malformations may follow the development of a double lumen within the endoderm of the developing bowel. The splanchnic mesoderm tends to condense around both elements to give a variable degree of *intestinal duplication.* In similar fashion a *solitary diverticulum* may arise, perhaps to become sequestered within the mesentery as an *enteric cyst.*

INTESTINE

In 2% of subjects a short, blind pocket projects from the antimesenteric aspect of the ileum, some two feet from the ileocolic junction. This is *Meckel's diverticulum;* its presence denotes persistence of the proximal end of the vitelline duct. The epithelium of Meckel's diverticulum has the curious property of differentiating at times into gastric mucous membrane or pancreatic acini.

Degrees of persistence of the vitelline duct are variable. A remnant of the duct or of a vitelline vessel may persist as a fibrous cord passing across the peritoneal cavity from ileum to umbilicus. Coils of intestine may loop around the cord and become obstructed at any time in postnatal life.

Fixation of the ascending and descending portions of the colon to the posterior abdominal wall may be faulty. Total failure, which is rare, is associated with persistence of the lower dorsal mesentery. The abnormal mobility of the colon may lead to torsion of the entire intestine around the mesenteric root with resultant strangulation of the intestinal vessels; the condition is known as *volvulus.* Partial failure of fixation is restricted to the proximal colon. The ascending colon may have a short mesentery, and the cecum may be unattached to the posterior abdominal wall (*mobile cecum*).

CECUM AND APPENDIX

The clinician will be faced with diagnostic difficulties should inflammation develop in an ectopic appendix, *i.e.,* one lying outside the right iliac fossa. The cause of the ectopia may be adhesion of the cecum to the visceral surface of the liver during fetal life (*subhepatic appendix*). A less common cause is *malrotation of the midgut,* the cecum and ascending colon lying in the center of the abdomen or even in the left lumbar or iliac regions.

A *fetal (infantile) cecum* is one whose neonatal form persists into adult life.

An infant who fails to excrete meconium may be found to have an *imperforate anus—*

an anal pit which ends blindly without communicating with the rectum. In such cases development of the lower part of the rectum has usually failed, and a fistula (opening) may occur between rectum and urethra or (in females) between rectum and vagina. Rarely, the fault is due merely to persistence of the anal membrane.

PANCREAS

The ventral pancreatic outgrowth may be double. In migrating to join the dorsal pancreatic outgrowth, one ventral bud may pass on each side of the gut, thereby giving rise to the condition of *annular pancreas.* Rarely, this malformation may cause duodenal obstruction.

KIDNEYS

Solitary kidney is sufficiently common (0.1% of the population) to require exclusion whenever surgical removal of a diseased kidney is contemplated. The cause may lie in failure of development of the ureteric bud or of the mesonephric duct from which it arises. In the latter case the ductus deferens (in males) is absent on the affected side.

Congenital cystic kidneys (*polycystic kidneys*) are found in about 0.2% of autopsy subjects (Fig. 11-33A). They are an important cause of renal failure. The kidneys, which are riddled with cysts, may become so large before birth as to obstruct the course of labor; or they may remain undetected until renal insufficiency sets in during adult life. The cause is uncertain. Although failure of union of the two elements—secretory and collecting—of the tubular system has been held responsible, it has been shown that many of the cysts do communicate with the collecting system, and that the related nephrons show no evidence of back pressure. The condition may also be associated with cyst formation in the pancreas, liver, and lungs, suggesting a more subtle growth defect of the mesoderm.

The metanephric blastemas are about 0.2 mm apart when they first appear. They may fuse at their lower poles to produce *horseshoe kidney.* Ascent of a horseshoe kidney is arrested by the inferior mesenteric artery (Fig. 11-33B). Medial rotation also fails, the renal pelves being directed anteriorly.

One or both kidneys may fail to ascend during the fetal period, retaining a blood supply from the iliac vessels.

FIG. 11-33. **A.** Congenital cystic kidney. (From a drawing by Mrs. H. Thelen.) **B.** Horseshoe kidney.

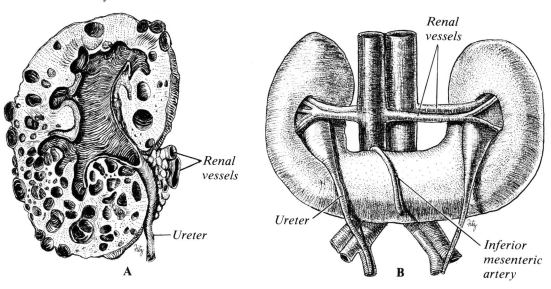

Following normal ascent of the kidney, a second, *aberrant* renal artery may pass from the aorta to the lower pole. Such a vessel may obstruct the ureter and cause *hydronephrosis, i.e.,* distension of the collecting system.

TESTES

Abnormalities of testicular descent are of two kinds. 1) In *maldescent* the organ is arrested somewhere along its normal pathway. *Cryptorchism* (*cryptos,* hidden) signifies retention of the testes within the abdomen, where normal spermatogenesis usually fails. In lesser degrees of maldescent the testis may lie anywhere along the inguinal canal. 2) In the condition known as *ectopia testis* the organ has taken up a position away from the normal pathway of descent. The lower end of the normal gubernaculum has a frayed arrangement; the bulk of its fibers occupy the scrotum but several strands pass to neighboring areas. In ectopia, the testis is thought to have followed one of these strands. The ectopic testis may be found on the lower abdominal wall, in the perineum, or in the upper part of the thigh.

Failure of closure of the processus vaginalis is common. Total failure provides the important *congenital hernial sac* into which loops of intestine readily protrude during fetal life or infancy (Fig. 11-34A). Occlusion at the lower end, with patency above, gives rise to the so-called *infantile hernial sac* (Fig. 11-34B); in the reverse condition the serous sac is sealed off from the general peritoneal cavity, but fluid accumulates within it to form an *infantile hydocele* (Fig. 11-34C). In another variant the sac is sealed above and below, becoming distended between to form an *encysted hydocele of the spermatic cord* (Fig. 11-34D).

UTERUS AND VAGINA

A variety of malformations of the uterus and vagina is possible, representing varying degrees of failure of union of the paramesonephric ducts. *Arcuate uterus,* resulting from arrest of the normal upward growth of the fundus, occurs in about 2% of females. Pregnancy in a uterus of this shape tends to result in an abnormal position of the fetus. The other end of the spectrum is represented by the very rare *uterus didelphys* (Gr., *delphys,* womb), in which total separation of the paramesonephric ducts leads to the formation of two vaginal plates, and hence to duplication of vagina as well as of uterus.

FIG. 11-34. **A.** Congenital hernial sac.
B. Infantile hernial sac.
C. Congenital hydrocele.
D. Encysted hydrocele of the spermatic cord.

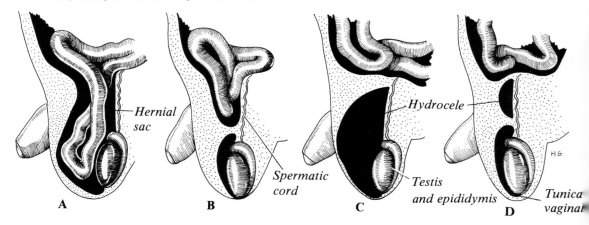

Imperforate hymen results from failure of the canalized vaginal plate to rupture into the vestibule. It manifests itself in the accumulation of menstrual blood within the vagina at puberty (*cryptomenorrhea*).

URETHRA

In *hypospadias,* there is an opening through the floor of the urethra, and the normal external meatus is absent. The condition is found at birth in 0.2% of males. It results from 1) failure of canalization of the ectodermal ingrowth that normally forms the glandular portion of the urethra; and 2) partial or complete failure of union of the urogenital folds. According to the position of the urinary meatus, hypospadias is classified as glandular, penile, scrotal, or perineal.

In *phimosis* the collarlike prepuce is too narrow, and it obstructs the urinary outlet. Manual retraction of a narrow prepuce is likely to result in compression of the penile urethra (*paraphimosis*).

SEXUAL ABNORMALITIES

A *true hermophrodite* is an individual who possesses both testicular and ovarian tissue. The condition is extremely rare, only about 150 cases having been proven. A uterus and vagina are present. The external genitalia may be either male or female in type. The cause is unknown.

A *pseudohermaphrodite* is an individual whose phenotypic sex, *i.e.,* sexual appearance, is at variance with his or her genotype. Female pseudohermaphrodites are of female genotype, but of male appearance. The commonest cause is congenital suprarenal cortical hyperplasia (already referred to). Male pseudohermaphrodites have a normal male genotype, but are of female appearance. The testes are undescended and there is a shallow vagina (but no uterus or oviducts). There is a familial tendency.

Various abnormalities of the external genitalia may be associated with abnormal karyotypes resulting from nondisjunction of the chromosomes during gametogenesis in one or other parent.

INFERIOR VENA CAVA

Anomalous development of the inferior vena cava is to be expected in view of its composite origin. The commonest deviations occur in the renal and postrenal parts, derived as they are from three paired channels. They do not give rise to clinical disorders.

SUGGESTED READING

Bulmer D: The development of the human vagina. J Anat 91:490–509, 1957

Du Bois AM: The embryonic kidney. In Rouiller C, Muller AF (eds): The Kidney. New York, Academic Press, 1968, pp 1–60

Elias H, Sherrick JC: Development of the human liver. In Morphology of the Liver. New York, Academic Press, 1969, pp 233–264

FitzGerald MJT, Nolan JP, O'Neill MN: The position of the human caecum in fetal life. J Anat 109:71–74, 1971

Fujimoto T, Miyayama Y, Fuyuta M: The origin, migration and fine morphology of human primordial germ cells. Anat Rec 188:315–330, 1977

Glenister TW: A correlation of the normal and abnormal development of the penile urethra and of the infra-umbilical abdominal wall. Br J Urol 30:117–126, 1958

Grobstein C: Inductive interaction in the development of the mouse metanephros. J Exp Zool 130:319–340, 1955

Jones HW: Development of the genitalia. In Barnes AC (ed): Intrauterine Development. Philadelphia, Lea & Febiger, 1968, pp 253–272

Kanagesuntheram R: Development of the human lesser sac. J Anat 91:188–206, 1957

Lauge–Hansen N: The mesenteries of the gastrointestinal tract. In The Development and the Embryological Anatomy of the Human Gastrointestinal Tract. Eindoven, Centrex Publishing, 1960, pp 57–68

Price JM, Donahoe PK, Ito Y, Hendren III WH: Programmed cell death in the müllerian duct induced by müllerian inhibiting substance. Am J Anat 149:353–376, 1977

Santulli TV, Amoury RA: Congenital anomalies of the gastrointestinal tract. Pediat Clin North Am 14:21–45, 1967

Sellmann AH, Dougherty CM: The development of the female genital tract. Ann NY Acad Sci 142:576–585, 1967

Shrock P: The processus vaginalis and gubernaculum. Surg Clin North Am 51:1263–1268, 1971

Wessels NK, Cohen JH: Early pancreas organogenesis: tissue interactions and mass effects. Dev Biol 15:237–270, 1967

Witschi E: Migrations of the germ cells of human embryos from the yolk sac to the primitive gonadal folds. Contrib Embryol Carnegie Inst 32:67–80, 1948

Chapter 12

head and neck

It has been seen in Chapter 6 that a series of branchial (pharyngeal) arches enclose the sides and floor of the primitive pharynx, and that the developing brain receives a diffuse investment from the cranial, unsegmented part of the mesoderm. The diffuse mesoderm, which for convenience we shall call the *head mesenchyme,* is the forerunner of the skull and upper part of the face. The branchial arch mesoderm gives rise to the lower part of the face, to the jaws and palate, and to the larynx and pharynx. The musculature of the head is derived both from pharyngeal arch mesoderm and from myotomes located in the head region. The covering ectoderm assists in the formation of skin, teeth, and glands, and contributes to the special senses and to sensory ganglia of the cranial nerves.

BRAIN

While flexion of the embryo is taking place during the somite period, closure of the neural groove proceeds quickly. The anterior neuropore closes on the 24th day after fertilization. The brain plate shows three serial expansions (Fig. 12-1) which are converted into vesicles by the closure of the neural folds. They are the *forebrain vesicle* (or *prosencephalon*), the *midbrain vesicle* (or *mesencephalon*), and the *hindbrain vesicle* (or *rhombencephalon*). The optic sulcus deepens to form the *optic vesicle,* attached to the prosencephalon by the hollow *optic stalk.* The optic vesicle induces a circumscribed thickening of the overlying ectoderm, the *lens placode* (Fig. 12-2).

The neural crest extends to the level of the mesencephalon. It gives rise to the ganglionic and neurolemmal cells of the cranial nerves and possibly to the pia-arachnoid surrounding the brain. Surprisingly, it also contributes precartilage cells to the mesoderm of the pharyngeal arches.

THE BRAIN FLEXURES

Development of the head fold imparts a *cervical flexure* to the neural tube, at the junction of rhombencephalon and spinal cord. A second *cephalic flexure* places the mesencephalon at the cephalic extremity of the embryo (Figs. 12-1C and 12-4)—a position that it maintains until submerged by the burgeoning cerebral hemispheres. The rhombencephalon buckles to create a third *pontine flexure.* The part of the rhombencephalon rostral to the pontine

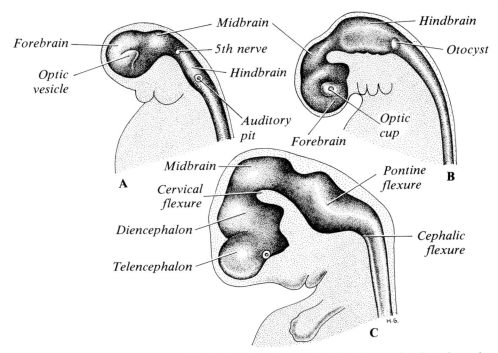

FIG. 12-1. Vesicles and flexures of the brain: **A,** at four weeks; **B,** at five weeks; **C,** at six weeks. (Adapted from Hochstetter F: Beitrage zur Entwicklungsgeschichte des menschlichen Gehirns. Vienna, Deuticke, 1929)

FIG. 12-2. Coronal section of the brain at four and one-half weeks. (Carnegie Collection) (x95)

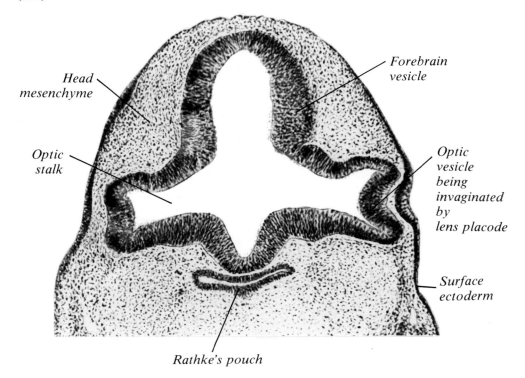

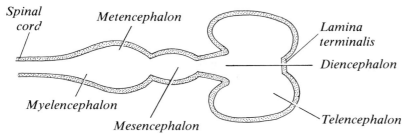

FIG. 12-3. Diagram of the cerebral vesicles.

flexure forms the pons and cerebellum; it is called the *metencephalon.* The part caudal to the flexure will form the medulla oblongata; this is called the *myelencephalon* (Fig. 12-3).

In the fifth week the prosencephalon gives rise to the paired *cerebral vesicles,* which constitute the *telencephalon.* The remaining, median portion of the prosencephalon constitutes the *diencephalon.* The anterior boundary of the diencephalon, representing the site of closure of the anterior neuropore, is the *lamina terminalis* (Fig. 12-3).

CEREBRAL COMMISSURES

The commissures connect like areas in the two cerebral hemispheres. The lamina terminalis is utilized by three major commissures. The first to appear is the *anterior commissure,* which initially connects the two olfactory bulbs; later, other fibers pass through the anterior commissure to connect the temporal lobes. The hippocampus is linked to its opposite number by the *fornix.* As development proceeds the fornix becomes the efferent tract from each hippocampus to the hypothalamus of its own side. The third commissure is the *corpus callosum,* which radiates throughout the cerebral cortex on each side. The small *posterior* and *habenular commissures* develop in relation to the pineal gland.

The lateral ventricles are invaginated by vascular pia mater, forming the *choroidal fissure.* The commissures enlarge rapidly to keep pace with the hemispheres, and the fornix and corpus callosum pass above the choroidal fissure, placing a second layer of pia mater on top of the choroidal vessels in the midline and forming a new roof for the third ventricle (Fig. 12-5). The double layer of pia, with its contained vessels, is the *velum interpositum.*

Between the corpus callosum and the fornix the wall of the hemisphere becomes stretched and thin, forming the *septum pellucidum.* The two septa fuse in the midline; the *cavum septi pellucidi,* when present, is a remnant of the interval between the two hemispheres in this area.

INTERNAL STRUCTURE

The structure of the developing brain is the same as that of the spinal cord, comprising ventricular, intermediate and marginal zones, together with thin roof and floor plates. The sulcus limitans can be traced upwards to the junction of mesencephalon with diencephalon; from here a shallow *hypothalamic sulcus* extends to the lamina terminalis (Fig. 12-5A). The nuclei of the thalamus develop in the mantle zone above the sulcus; the hypothalamic nuclei develop below it. Because the latter do not give rise to peripheral nerves they are not considered to be homologous with the neurons of the basal plate.

The pontine flexure causes the alar laminae to flare outwards so that the roof plate becomes diamond-shaped. The central canal is thereby enlarged to form the *fourth ventricle.* A transverse section through metencephalon or upper myelencephalon shows the alar plate to be lateral to, rather than behind, the sulcus limitans (Fig. 12-6).

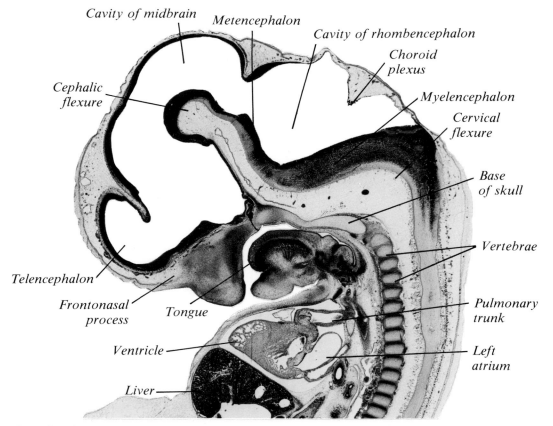

FIG. 12-4. Sagittal section of head and thorax at six weeks. (Carnegie Collection) (x18)

FIG. 12-5. Diagrams of stages in the development of the three major cerebral commissures.

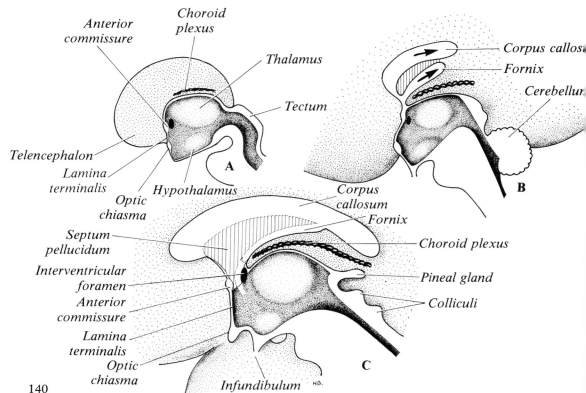

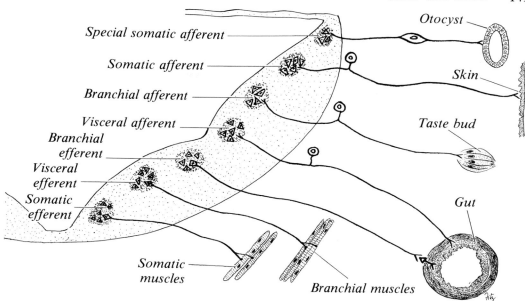

FIG. 12-6. Diagram of the efferent and afferent cell columns in the hindbrain.

BASAL PLATE IN THE BRAIN STEM

It will be seen later in this chapter that the striated muscle of the head region has two sources. 1) The muscles of the tongue and the extrinsic muscles of the eye develop from myotomes. 2) The muscles of the face, jaws, larynx, and pharynx develop from the branchial arches. The nuclear groups innervating the striated muscle of eye and tongue are called *somatic efferent* because they are homologous with the motoneurons of the ventral gray matter of the spinal cord, which supply the musculature of the body wall (or *soma*). The nuclei concerned are those of the oculomotor, trochlear, and abducent nerves (to the eye) and the hypoglossal nerve (to the tongue). The nuclei supplying muscles of the branchial arch origin are the motor nucleus of the trigeminal (to the muscles of mastication), facial (to the facial muscles), and the nucleus ambiguus which supplies the laryngeal and pharyngeal muscles by way of the glossopharyngeal and vagus nerves.

The branchial efferent cell column lies between the somatic efferent and *visceral efferent* column (Fig. 12-6). The visceral efferent column in the brain stem is homologous with the sympathetic preganglionic column in the spinal cord; it comprises the nuclei of origin of the parasympathetic component of certain cranial nerves—the Edinger–Westphal nucleus in the midbrain (to the sphincter pupillae and ciliary muscle of the eye), the salivary nuclei in the pons (to the lacrimal, submandibular, and parotid glands), and the dorsal motor nucleus of the vagus in the medulla oblongata.

ALAR PLATE IN THE BRAIN STEM

The most medial cell group is the (general) *visceral afferent* column, formed by the dorsal sensory nucleus of the vagus. Lateral to this is the *branchial* (or *special visceral*) afferent column, represented by the nucleus of the *tractus solitarius,* which receives taste fibers from the tongue and palate by way of the nervus intermedius and the glossopharyngeal and vagus nerves.

The *somatic afferent* column has a double representation in the brain stem. The *general somatic afferent* column is formed by the nuclei of termination of the trigeminal sensory neurons. The *special somatic afferent* column occupies the margin of the alar lamina in the myelencephalon. It comprises the cochlear and vestibular nuclei, which receive the special sensory afferents from the inner ear.

The nuclear masses that come to occupy the brain stem at some distance from the central gray matter—*red nucleus, substantia nigra, colliculi, olive,* and *gracile* and *cuneate nuclei*—are thought to arise from the regional alar lamina and to migrate into the marginal layer. In the midbrain the several nuclear masses compress the central canal so that it becomes the narrow *aqueduct.* The *nuclei pontis,* together with the massive corticoponticerebellar system that later occupies the marginal zone, obliterate the pontine flexure.

CEREBELLUM

Phylogenetically, the cerebellum consists of three parts: the *archicerebellum,* receiving connections from the vestibular nuclei; the *paleocerebellum,* with afferents from the spinocerebellar tracts; and the *neocerebellum,* linked to the cerebral cortex. Experimental work has shown that the connections of the cerebellum cannot be entirely accounted for by its phylogeny. The paleocerebellum, for example, receives a substantial input from several parts of the cerebral cortex.

In the metencephalon the margins of the flared alar laminae curl inwards to form the *rhombic lip.* Here neuroblasts form bilateral swellings that fuse in the midline to produce the *cerebellar primordium* (Fig. 12-7A). The early enlargement of the cerebellum is inwards, and the fourth ventricle is largely filled (Fig. 12-8); the so-called "eversion" of the organ is the result of the later rapid growth of the extraventricular portion (Fig. 12-7B).

The first part to differentiate is the *archicerebellum,* which phylogenetically is the oldest and is richly connected to the vestibular nerve. It comprises the *nodule and flocculus* (Fig. 12-7B), which are later dwarfed by the expansion of the cerebellar hemispheres.

The remainder of the cerebellum has been traditionally divided into the *paleocerebellum* (with spinal connections) and the *neocerebellum* (with cerebral connections). However, this division is of little functional value because of the development of extensive overlaps of spinal and cerebral connections within the cerebellar cortex.

The cerebellar cortex is formed by the migration of precursor cells from the ventricular zone outwards into the marginal zone. Two successive migrations take place, and the histodifferentiation of the cortex into molecular, Purkinje, and granular layers is extremely complex and continues into the postnatal period. The *dentate* and other deep nuclei are formed by the maturation of neuroblasts that do not migrate outside the intermediate zone.

FIG. 12-7. The hindbrain with roof plate cut away. **A,** at eight weeks; **B,** at 12 weeks. (Adapted from Streeter GL: in Keibel F, Mall FP (eds): Manual of Human Embryology. Philadelphia, JB Lippincott, 1910, p 60 [Figs 44 and 45])

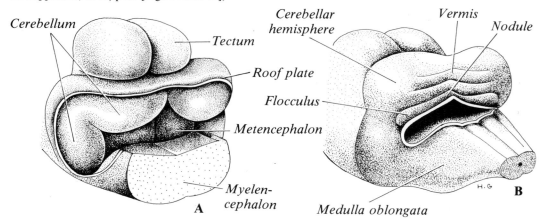

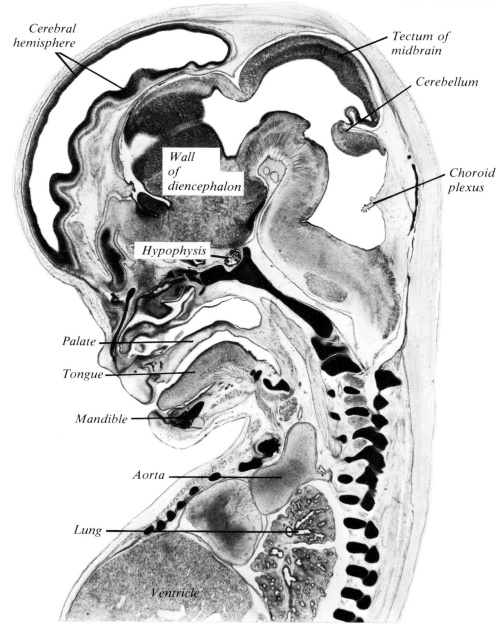

Cerebral
hemisphere

Tectum of
midbrain

Cerebellum

Wall
of
diencephalon

Choroid
plexus

Hypophysis

Palate

Tongue

Mandible

Aorta

Lung

Ventricle

FIG. 12-8. Sagittal section of head and thorax at 10 weeks. (Carnegie Collection) (x6)

In the fourth month the median and lateral apertures of the ventricle appear by the formation and rupture of three roof-plate diverticuli.

DIENCEPHALON

In the absence of a definable basal plate, the diencephalon is considered to be made up of a roof plate and of two alar plates that meet in its floor. Three nuclear masses develop in the lateral wall of the diencephalon—the *epithalamus,* the *thalamus,* and the *hypothalamus.* The cerebral vesicles develop in the interval between the thalamus and the lamina terminalis.

The epithalamus gives rise to the *pineal gland* and to the *habenular nucleus.* The thalamus appears in the form of six nuclear groups—anterior, ventral, medial, and lateral, together with the *medial and lateral geniculate bodies*. The enlarging thalami compress the cavity of the diencephalon until it becomes the slitlike *third ventricle* (Fig. 12-9). The anterior wall of the hypothalamus is invaded by the *optic chiasma* (Fig. 12-5). The floor of the hypothalamus gives rise to the *infundibulum,* which is the primordium of the neurohypophysis, and to the *mammillary bodies*.

TELENCEPHALON

The telencephalon comprises the paired cerebral vesicles and the lamina terminalis between them. The forebrain cavity extends into the vesicles, forming the *lateral ventricles,* which communicate with the third ventricle through the *interventricular foramen.*

The cerebral vesicles give rise to the *cerebral hemispheres.* The most primitive parts of the hemispheres are the first to appear; these parts lag behind during later growth, and the phylogenetically more advanced parts of the brain either distort them by stretching and attenuation, or are themselves distorted through anchorage to relatively immobile cell masses. Thus the olfactory region, or *rhinencephalon,* which dominates the brain of lower vertebrates, becomes stretched and partly obliterated by subsequent growth of the hemisphere; and the *corpus striatum,* dominant in the reptile, comes to form half of the bulk of the early human brain; then it falters, forming a relatively stable pivot around which the expanding hemisphere rotates.

As each cerebral vesicle expands into the surrounding mesoderm, neuroblasts congregate in its lower half to form the *corpus striatum* (Fig. 12-9A). The upper half of each vesicle

FIG. 12-9. Stages in the development of the cerebral hemispheres: **A,** at seven weeks; **B,** at 17 weeks; **C,** adult. (Adapted from Hochstetter F: Beitrage zur Entwicklungsgeschichte des menschlichen Gehirns. Vienna, Deuticke, 1929)

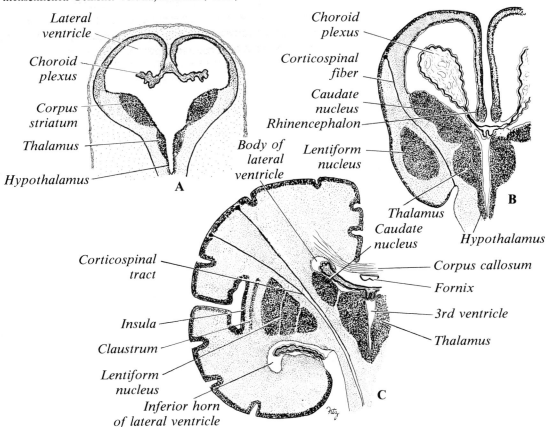

enlarges upwards and medially, compressing the intervening mesoderm to form the *falx cerebri*. In the sagittal plane the vesicles extend in an arch around the corpus striatum. The *temporal lobes* are formed by forward extension below the level of the corpus striatum. Later, the *occipital lobes* arise as blunt backward projections.

After the 12th week the rate of growth of the corpus striatum declines; it sinks beneath the surface, drawing with it a laminar piece of gray matter called the *claustrum*. The cortex that later differentiates external to the claustrum appears to be inhibited in its growth; it is overlapped by the frontal, parietal, and temporal lobes of the brain, and remains as the sunken *insula* (Fig. 12-9C).

The deep gutter between temporal lobe and diencephalon is filled by thickening of the walls of the interventricular foramen—a prerequisite for the passage of the great motor and sensory pathways. These fiber systems pursue the shortest course between cerebral cortex and brain stem; they cleave the corpus striatum into two parts, creating the *internal capsule* between them. The medial part of the corpus striatum is the *caudate nucleus,* the lateral part is the *lentiform nucleus* (Fig. 12-9B and C).

CEREBRAL CORTEX

The expanding cerebral vesicles display the same histologic structure as the neural tube elsewhere, with ventricular, intermediate, and marginal zones. The laminated gray matter of the cerebral cortex is constructed by the outward migration of germinal cells. One of the puzzles concerning cortical development has been the knowledge that the earliest (and phylogenetically oldest) layers of cortical neurons come to occupy the deepest part of the adult cortex (closest to the ventricle); the later layers take up progressively more superficial positions, having apparently migrated through the deeper laminae. Recent work has shown that the individual germinal (ependymal) cells extend from the inner to the outer

FIG. 12-10. Scheme to show development of nerve cells in the cerebral cortex: **A**, mitosis in ventricular zone; **B**, migration of nucleus of cell 1; **C**, nucleus of cell 1 approaching pial surface; **D**, extrusion of cell 1, mitosis in ventricular zone; **E**, differentiation of cell 1, migration of nucleus 2; **F**, repetition of C; **G**, extrusion of cell 2 superficial to cell 1. (Adapted from Berry M and Rogers AW: J Anat 99:691, 1965)

Pial surface

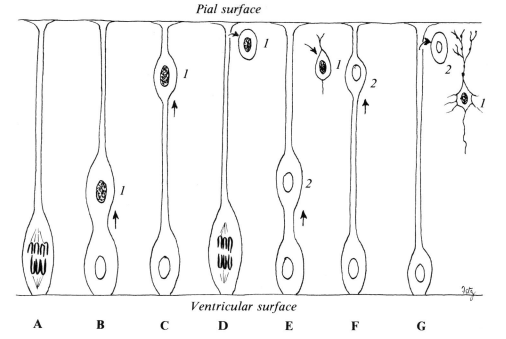

Ventricular surface

A   B   C   D   E   F   G

limiting membranes, *i.e.,* from ventricular to pial surfaces. Nuclear division takes place in the ventricular zone (Fig. 12-10). One daughter nucleus remains in the ventricular zone while the second moves outwards within the ribbon of cytoplasm. Only when it reaches the marginal zone does it separate from the parent cell, the nucleus being extruded here in a droplet of cytoplasm. This newly formed neuroblast gives rise to apical and basal dendrites and an axon, adopting the typical pyramidal shape of cortical neurons while receding from the pial surface along a scaffolding of neuroglial cells. The germinal cells maintain their attachment to the limiting membranes, and the later outward migration of daughter nuclei takes place as before. These nuclei likewise are detached from the parent cell close to the outer limiting membrane, and accordingly occupy a more superficial position in the cortex.

When development of the brain is considered as a whole, three phases can be observed: 1) the production of neuroblasts, during the 4th to 20th weeks; 2) multiplication of gliablasts, commencing at about the 20th week and continuing until well into the second postnatal year; and 3) maturation of neurons, characterized by the prodigious growth of dendritic trees within the gray matter, and by myelination of axons by oligodendrocytes in the white matter. The third component is mainly responsible for the *brain growth spurt,* a term used to define the period of most rapid increase in brain size. Determinations of whole brain weights show that the velocity of brain growth is greatest during the last 10 prenatal weeks and the first 20 postnatal weeks (Fig. 12-11). Although the rate of growth diminishes later on, the brain more than doubles its weight during the first postnatal year, and achieves 90% of its adult size by the end of the sixth year.

Infants born in deprived conditions to emaciated mothers show a remarkably normal degree of brain development. During the first two postnatal years an adequate calorie intake is, however, *crucial* for the rapid growth of neuronal dendritic trees, proliferation of synaptic contacts, and myelination of axons. Millions of children become mentally retarded each year because this support is not forthcoming.

FIG. 12-11. Growth velocity and weight curves for the human brain. (Adapted from Dobbins J: in Davis JA, Dobbing J [eds]: Scientific Foundations of Pediatrics. London, Heinemann, 1975, pp 565–576)

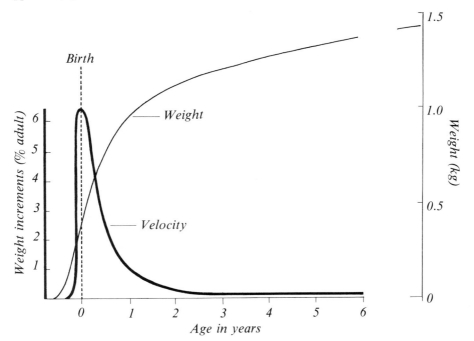

GYRI AND SULCI

Until the 16th week the surface of the brain is quite smooth. Thereafter, growth of the cortex outstrips that of the underlying white matter so that *convolutions (gyri)* appear, with *sulci* between.

THE SKULL

BASE

At the close of the second month, chondrogenesis is proceeding rapidly in the mesoderm below the brain. A single median cartilaginous plate surrounds the notochord and extends forwards on each side of the pituitary gland. It is flanked by four paired lateral centers of chondrification; the cranial nerves and vessels occupy the intervals between the nine cartilaginous islands.

The median cartilaginous plate consists of six elements—*occipital sclerotomes;* the *parachordal cartilage,* surrounding the tip of the notochord; and the small, paired *hypophyseal* and *trabecular cartilages* (Fig. 12-12A). The occipital sclerotomes arise from four *occipital somites* that are in series with the cervical somites. Their pre-muscle element gives rise to the muscles of the tongue. The sclerotomes blend around the notochord and send a broad neural arch to surround the neural tube (Fig. 12-12B). They form the part of the occipital bone which surrounds the foramen magnum (Fig. 12-12C). The parachordal cartilage gives rise to the basiocciput, and the hypophyseal cartilages give rise to the body of

FIG. 12-12. Scheme to show development of the skull, with incorporation of the cranial nerves.

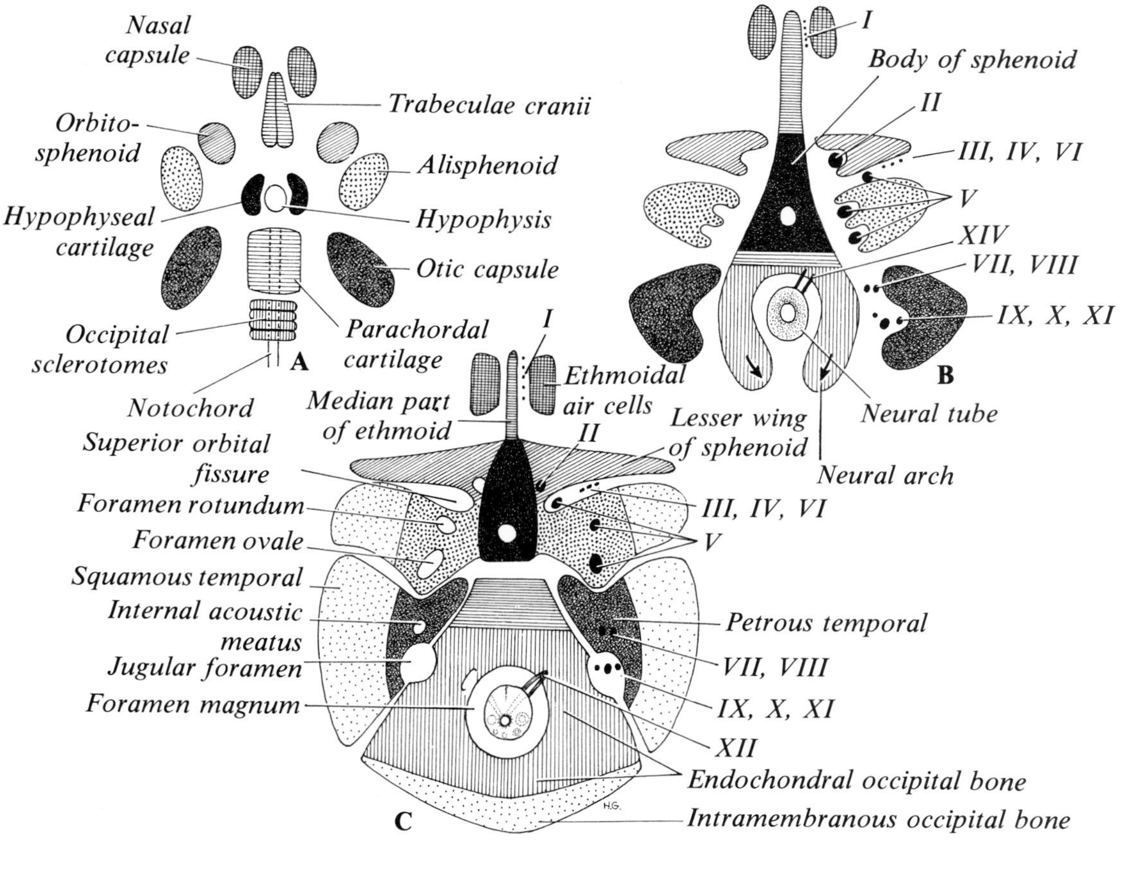

sphenoid bone. The vertical part of the ethmoid (*crista galli* and *perpendicular plate*) is derived from the fused trabeculae cranii.

The lateral cartilaginous centers are the *nasal capsules,* the *orbitosphenoids,* the *alisphenoids,* and the *otic capsules* (Fig. 12-12A). The nasal capsules form the lateral part of the ethmoid bone, which encloses the ethmoidal air cells. The orbitosphenoid is the precursor of the lesser wing of the sphenoid bone. It approaches the median cartilaginous plate, dividing to enclose the optic nerve (Fig. 12-12B). The alisphenoid is the precursor of the inner part of the greater wing of the sphenoid bone. It is indented by the maxillary and mandibular nerves (Fig. 12-12B), and these come to be enclosed by its medial growth (Fig. 12-12C). The gap between orbitosphenoid and alisphenoid narrows to become the *superior orbital fissure* (Fig. 12-12C). The otic capsule is a cartilaginous shell surrounding the otocyst (see section "Inner Ear"). It forms the *petrous temporal* bone, also the *mastoid process* which grows down from the petrous part after birth. The petrous temporal bone is pierced by the facial and vestibulocochlear nerves. The facial nerve, on its emergence from the temporal bone, is unprotected because of the late development of the mastoid process. Not infrequently it is temporarily paralyzed by pressure of the obstetrician's forceps during a difficult delivery.

The anterior cardinal vein and the ninth, tenth, and eleventh cranial nerves indent the adjacent edges of the petrous temporal and occipital bones, creating the *jugular foramen* (Fig. 12-12C).

Two parts of the temporal bone—the petromastoid and the styloid process—have cartilaginous precursors, and two—the squamous and the tympanic plate—ossify in membrane. At the time of birth the tympanic part is represented by the horseshoe-shaped *tympanic ring* (Fig. 12-13A), from which the *tympanic plate* grows laterally to form the bony floor of the external acoustic meatus close to the tympanic membrane.

VAULT

Intramembranous ossification commences in the third month from single centers in the parietal, sphenoid (outer part of greater wing), temporal (squamous part), and occipital (interparietal part) regions. The frontal bone develops from two centers, and the two plates of bone fuse in the midline. Fusion is incomplete at birth, so that the *anterior fontanelle* is diamond-shaped (Fig. 12-13). This area, clinically important for the assessment of intracranial pressure, is palpable for 18 months after birth and closes completely at about two years. The smaller *posterior fontanelle* closes a year earlier.

The *frontal and parietal eminences* mark the site of the respective centers of ossification. They are prominent in the skull of the newborn (Fig. 12-12) and they persist throughout life.

FIG. 12-13. The skull at birth: **A,** from the left side; **B,** from above.

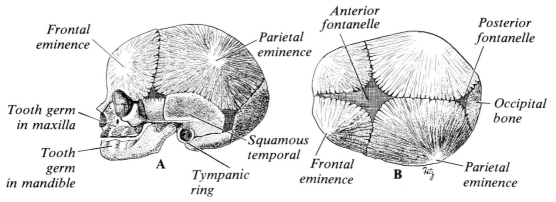

SPLANCHNOCRANIUM

The light bones of the face—maxillas, premaxillas, zygomatics, lacrimals, palatines, and nasals—ossify from single centers. The mandible is considered later.

The derivation of the principal parts of the skull is summarized in Table 12-1.

TABLE 12-1. DERIVATON OF SKULL BONES

BONE	OSSIFICATION	PRECURSOR
Parietal	Membrane	Head mesenchyme
Frontal	Membrane	Head mesenchyme
Nasal	Membrane	Frontonasal process
Maxilla	Membrane	Maxillary process
Mandible	Membrane	Mandibular arch
Ethmoid (central part)	Cartilage	Trabeculae cranii
Ethmoid (labyrinth)	Cartilage	Nasal capsule
Sphenoid (body)	Cartilage	Hypophyseal cartilages
Sphenoid (lesser wing)	Cartilage	Orbitosphenoid
Sphenoid (inner part of greater wing)	Cartilage	Alisphenoid
Sphenoid (outer part of greater wing and pterygoid plates)	Membrane	Head mesenchyme
Temporal (petromastoid)	Cartilage	Otic capsule
Temporal (styloid process)	Cartilage	Hyoid arch
Temporal (squamous)	Membrane	Head mesenchyme
Temporal (tympanic plate)	Membrane	Head mesenchyme
Occipital (basilar part)	Cartilage	Parachordal cartilage
Occipital (around foramen magnum)	Cartilage	Occipital sclerotomes
Occipital (interparietal part)	Membrane	Head mesenchyme

HYPOPHYSIS

The hypophysis is entirely ectodermal in origin. The *anterior lobe (adenohypophysis)* is derived from the ectodermal roof of the stomodeum, the *posterior lobe (neurohypophysis)* from the floor of the diencephalon (Fig. 12-14).

At the end of the third week the anterior lobe arises as the hollow *Rathke's pouch* immediately external to the oral membrane. Three weeks later the posterior lobe grows down from the diencephalon. It is embraced by lateral expansions of Rathke's pouch. The stalk of the pouch normally disappears. The neural lobe retains its diencephalic connection, which forms the *infundibulum.*

The posterior wall of Rathke's pouch remains thin and forms the *middle lobe* of the hypophysis. The lumen of the pouch is usually obliterated in man. The posterior lobe gives

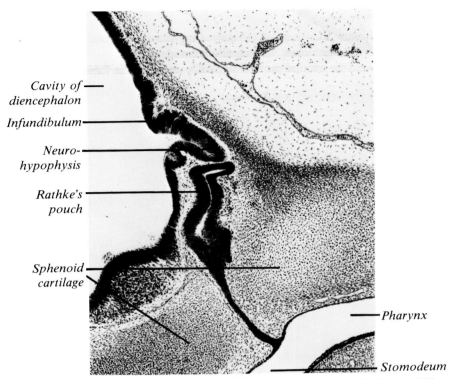

Cavity of — diencephalon

Infundibulum —

Neuro- hypophysis

Rathke's pouch

Sphenoid cartilage

Pharynx

Stomodeum

FIG. 12-14. Enlargement from the center of Figure 12-4. (Carnegie Collection) (x120)

rise to modified neuroglial cells, the *pituicytes*. From the hypothalamus, axons containing neurosecretory material grow down the infundibulum and permeate among them.

FATE OF THE BRANCHIAL ARCHES

The branchial arches bulge into the side walls of the foregut and, meeting each other in its floor, displace the heart caudally to establish the neck region of the embryo. Mammalian arches are six in number on each side, but in man the fifth is trivial in size and is transient. The ectodermal grooves between adjacent arches are called the *branchial clefts,* and the endodermal grooves the *branchial pouches.* The *embryonic pharynx* may be defined as the part of the foregut that has the branchial (pharyngeal) arches in its walls and floor (Fig. 12-15). It gives rise to the pharynx of the adult and, with the assistance of the stomodeum, to the oral cavity also.

The fate of the arches is diverse. Altogether they form the skeleton, musculature, and blood vessels of the jaws, palate, larynx, and pharynx, and the muscles of the face.

The dorsal end of each arch approaches the hindbrain; here it is invaded by nerve fibers from the branchial efferent cell column. The ventral ends converge upon the pericardium where they are accessible to the outflow channel from the heart—the truncus arteriosus. The truncus connects with capillaries differentiating within the arches, and these in turn become linked with the corresponding dorsal aortae (Fig. 6-9). Only three pairs of branchial arteries persist—the third, fourth, and sixth. Their fate is considered in Chapter 10.

FIRST BRANCHIAL ARCH

During the fifth and sixth weeks, fusion of the two first or mandibular arches in the midline is completed. The maxillary processes also come together at this time. The mandibular

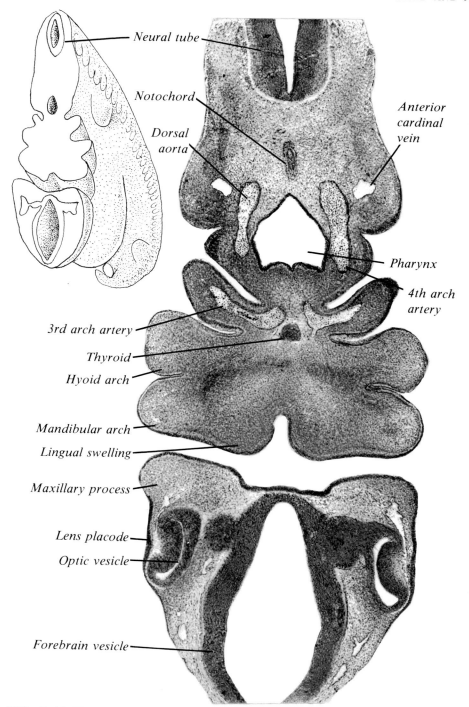

Neural tube

Notochord

Dorsal aorta

Anterior cardinal vein

Pharynx

4th arch artery

3rd arch artery

Thyroid

Hyoid arch

Mandibular arch

Lingual swelling

Maxillary process

Lens placode

Optic vesicle

Forebrain vesicle

FIG. 12-15. The inset shows the level of this section through the brain and branchial arches of an embryo in the fifth week. (Carnegie Collection) (x85)

arches give rise to two *lingual swellings* which enlarge and fuse to form the mesenchymal primordium of the anterior two-thirds of the tongue (Figs. 12-15 and 12-16). They also form a small, median *tuberculum impar,* but this soon regresses. The enlarging tongue rudiment becomes separated from the parent mesoderm by a deep *linguogingival groove,* which eventually frees the anterior part of the tongue from the mandible (Fig. 12-16C).

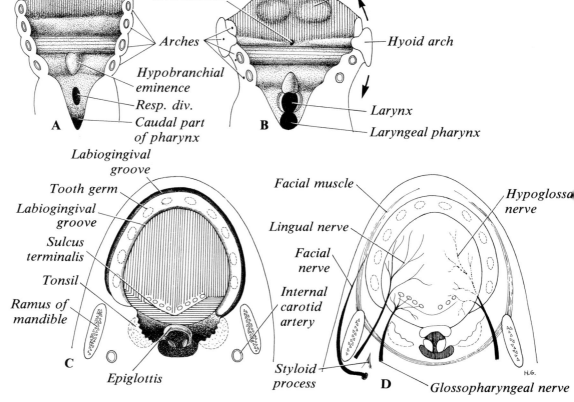

FIG. 12-16. **A.** The floor of the embryonic pharynx (resp. div., respiratory diverticulum).
B. Later stage showing outward migration **(arrows)** of the hyoid arch.
C. Connective tissue components of the tongue derived from the mandibular arch (vertical shading) and third arch (horizontal shading); the position of the tooth germs is indicated.
D. Innervation of the tongue and of the facial muscles; the circumvallate papillae are anterior to the sulcus terminalis.

A second *labiogingival groove* appears in the upper and lower jaws; it deepens to form the *vestibule of the mouth* and to define the gums (gingivae).

Beneath the lower gums the core of the first arch chondrifies on each side to form *Meckel's cartilage* (Fig. 12-19). The dorsal end of each is incorporated in the developing temporal bone and forms the upper parts of *malleus* and *incus*. In the region of the body of the mandible, Meckel's cartilages, together with the nerve and blood supply to the teeth, are imprisoned by successive plates of membrane bone derived from the surrounding mesoderm (Fig. 12-20). As the deposition of bone proceeds, the cartilage is resorbed; it contributes only a small amount of endochondral bone to the mandible near the midline.

The remarkable *condylar growth* center of the mandible appears in the fifth month. The mesenchyme in the condyle transforms into cartilage, which is continuously added to from the perichondrium on its upper surface. The proliferating cartilage is replaced by bone from below, in the usual way. The condylar center is responsible for the elongation of the mandibular ramus during the first ten years. In combination with molding of the anterior and posterior borders, its growth maintains the teeth in proper occlusive alignment during their eruption.

The *muscles of mastication* develop from the first arch mesoderm. The branchial efferent nerve to the muscles is the motor root of the trigeminal.

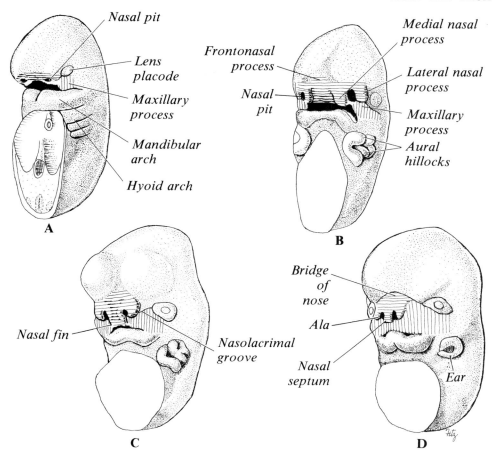

FIG. 12-17. Development of the face: **A,** early fifth week; **B,** early sixth week; **C,** late sixth week; **D,** seven weeks. **Vertical shading,** maxillary processes; **horizontal shading,** frontonasal process. (Adapted in part from class drawings by Pearson)

FIG. 12-18. Development of the palate: **A,** at six weeks (the **arrow** enters the anterior naris and emerges through the primitive posterior naris); **B,** at seven weeks; **C,** at 11 weeks (the **arrow** emerges through the definitive posterior naris). **FNP,** frontonasal process.

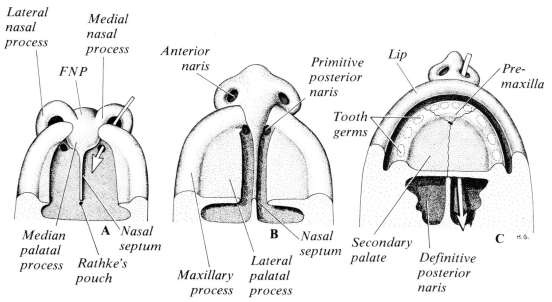

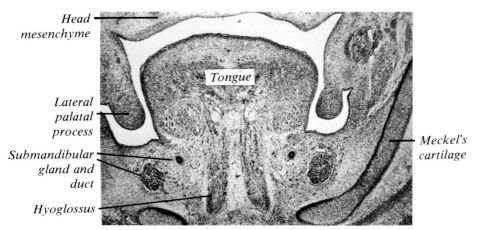

Head
mesenchyme

Tongue

Lateral
palatal
process

Submandibular
gland and
duct

Hyoglossus

Meckel's
cartilage

FIG. 12-19. Coronal section early in the eighth week, showing the lateral palatal processes beside the developing tongue. (Cambridge Collection) (x35)

FIG. 12-20. Coronal section late in the eighth week, showing the horizontal position of the lateral palatal processes, and the downgrowth of the nasal septum. (Cambridge Collection) (x12)

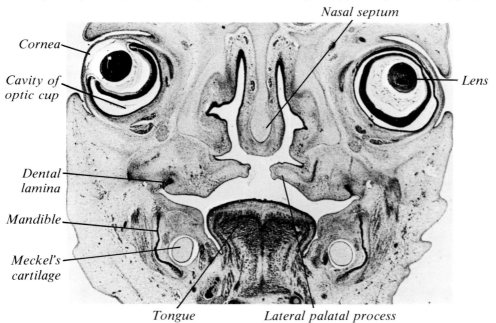

Nasal septum

Cornea

Cavity of
optic cup

Lens

Dental
lamina

Mandible

Meckel's
cartilage

Tongue   Lateral palatal process

SECOND BRANCHIAL ARCH

The two hyoid arches are characterized by a remarkable separation of their skeletal and muscular elements. The core of the conjoint hyoid arches forms a U-shaped cartilage whose middle section ossifies as the upper part of the *hyoid bone*. The dorsal end of the cartilage on each side is incorporated in the middle ear and forms the *stapes,* as well as the lower parts of malleus and incus. Below the ear it forms the *styloid process* of the temporal bone. Between the styloid process and hyoid bone the cartilage is lost, but its perichondrium persists as the *stylohyoid ligament.*

The muscular element of the hyoid arch migrates outside the mandibular arch and spreads, fanlike, to enclose almost the entire head and neck. It forms the *muscles of facial expression.* Only the *stapedius* and *stylohyoid* retain their connections to the arch skeleton. The *facial* is the branchial efferent nerve to the hyoid arch musculature.

THIRD TO SIXTH BRANCHIAL ARCHES

The third arch forms the mesenchymal primordium of the posterior one-third of the tongue. Its only muscular component is the *stylopharyngeus muscle.* Its cartilaginous element ossifies to form the lower part of the hyoid bone. The *glossopharyngeal* is the nerve of the third arch, the motor fibers arising in the nucleus ambiguus.

The fourth and sixth arches mingle as they produce the *cartilages* and *ligaments* of the *larynx,* the *intrinsic muscles of larynx and pharynx,* and the *levator palati.* The *vagus* nerve supplies all the muscles, by means of fibers that arise in the nucleus ambiguus.

The skeletal and muscular derivatives of the branchial arch mesoderm are summarized in Table 12-2; the nerves invading the arches are included.

TABLE 12-2. DERIVATIVES AND INNERVATION OF THE BRANCHIAL ARCHES

ARCH	SKELETAL DERIVATIVES	MUSCLES	INNERVATION
Mandibular	Mandible Maxilla Upper parts of malleus and incus	Muscles of mastication Tensor tympani Tensor palati	Mandibular nerve
Hyoid	Lower parts of malleus and incus Stapes Styloid process Stylohyoid ligament Upper part of hyoid bone	Muscles of facial expression Stapedius Stylohyoid	VII
Third	Lower part of hyoid bone	Stylopharyngeus	Nucleus ambiguus (IX)
Forth and sixth	Cartilages of larynx	Pharyngeal constrictors Intrinsic muscles of larynx Levator palati	Nucleus ambiguus (X)

FURTHER DEVELOPMENT OF THE TONGUE

The mesenchymal primordia of the tongue, laid down by the first and third arches, are nothing more than a scaffolding provided for the migration of pre-muscle tissue from the occipital myotomes. The function of the mesenchyme corresponds to that of the somatopleure which, in the trunk region, forms a substrate for the migration of somites into the body wall. The hypoglossal nerve innervates the occipital somites, and its nucleus has been seen to occupy the somatic efferent cell column in the medulla oblongata.

The epithelium covering the anterior two-thirds is supplied by the lingual branch of the mandibular nerve (Fig. 12-16D). Taste sensation here is mediated by the *chorda tympani* branch of the facial nerve. The epithelium of the posterior one-third is supplied by the *glossopharyngeal nerve,* both for common sensation and taste. The dividing line between the mandibular and hyoid arch components of the connective tissue of the tongue is the V-shaped *sulcus terminalis.* Surprisingly, the glossopharyngeal nerve overlaps the sulcus to supply the taste buds of the *vallate papillae* (Fig. 12-16D).

FATE OF THE BRANCHIAL CLEFTS

Only the first branchial cleft is normally of permanent significance. It forms the *external acoustic meatus* (see section "Outer Ear").

As the second arch extends down the neck (to form the platysma muscle sheet) it overlaps the second, third, and fourth branchial clefts. It fuses below with a mesodermal elevation, the *epipericardial ridge,* which lodges the anterior cardinal vein. The space so enclosed is the *cervical sinus.* It is normally obliterated.

FACE, PALATE, AND NOSE

An understanding of the development of the face and palate is of particular importance in view of the prevalence of malformations of the upper lip and palate.

THE FACE

The oral membrane ruptures before the end of the fourth week, throwing the pharynx into communication with the amniotic cavity. The ectoderm above the stomodeum thickens on each side to form the *nasal placodes.* Similar thickenings above the maxillary processes form the *lens placodes* (Fig. 12-17A). The mesoderm over the forebrain thickens a little to form the *frontonasal process* (Fig. 12-17B).

During the fifth week the nasal placodes recede into deepening *nasal pits.* The recession of the placodes is brought about by extension of the placodal epithelium into the underlying head mesenchyme, and by the heaping up of frontonasal mesoderm on each side of the placodes, as the *medial* and *lateral nasal processes.* The nasal pits form the *anterior nares,* or nostrils (Fig. 12-17B). The frontonasal process itself extends downwards beneath the ectoderm to form the bridge of the nose. Its lower end grows dorsally as the *median palatal process,* or *primary palate* (Fig. 12-18A). The medial nasal processes form the lower part of the nasal septum, between the nostrils. The lateral nasal processes form the *alae* of the nose (Fig. 12-17D).

Each nasal pit deepens to form a *nasal sac.* The placodal epithelium, now in the roof of the sac, differentiates to form the *olfactory epithelium.* The floor of the sac thins out the underlying roof of the stomodeum to form the *bucconasal membrane,* which ruptures to establish the *primitive posterior naris* (Fig. 12-18A, **arrow**).

A narrow strand of head mesenchyme connects the medial nasal process to the maxillary process below the nasal pit from the earliest stages (Fig. 12-17A and B). The maxillary process extends medially below the lateral nasal process and comes into full contact with the medial nasal process. The ectoderm on their contiguous surfaces forms the *nasal fin,* which extends from the anterior naris to the level of the connection between maxillary process and medial nasal process (Fig. 12-17C). During later development the mutual compression is reduced and the processes move apart, causing the nasal fin to disappear (Fig. 12-17D). Recent observations on human embryos suggest that mesodermal penetration of the nasal fin does not occur; instead the mesodermal connection below the fin expands to fill the entire interval between anterior naris and stomodeum (Fig. 12-17D).

The upper lip is defined by the development of the labiogingival sulcus of the upper jaw; this separates the lip from the palate all around.

The relative contributions of the frontonasal and maxillary processes to the formation of the upper lip is uncertain. Most workers consider that the maxillary processes meet one another in the midline to create the grooved *philtrum* of the upper lip. The innervation of the epithelial covering of the entire upper lip by the maxillary nerves offers indirect support for this concept. Others believe the philtrum to be derived from the frontonasal process.

The maxillary process meets the lateral nasal process along a line extending from the inner angle of the eye to the nostril. Along this line the ectoderm forms the deep *nasolacrimal groove* (Fig. 12-17C). The groove is later submerged by the adjacent mesoderm to form the *nasolacrimal duct,* which extends from the inner angle of the eye to the inferior meatus of the nose.

THE PALATE AND NOSE

The anterior part of the maxillary process fuses with the median palatine process or primary palate. It forms the *premaxilla;* this portion of the hard palate in the adult carries the incisor teeth (Fig. 12-18C).

Lateral palatal processes develop from the maxillary processes during the sixth week (Fig. 12-18). The lateral palatal processes hang down beside the tongue until the eighth week (Fig. 12-19); then they become horizontal (Fig. 12-20), grow across the upper surface of the tongue and fuse with one another before the end of the tenth week (Fig. 12-21). Their

FIG. 12-21. The insert shows the plane of this section through the nose, mouth, larynx, and pharynx at 11 weeks. (Carnegie Collection) (x18)

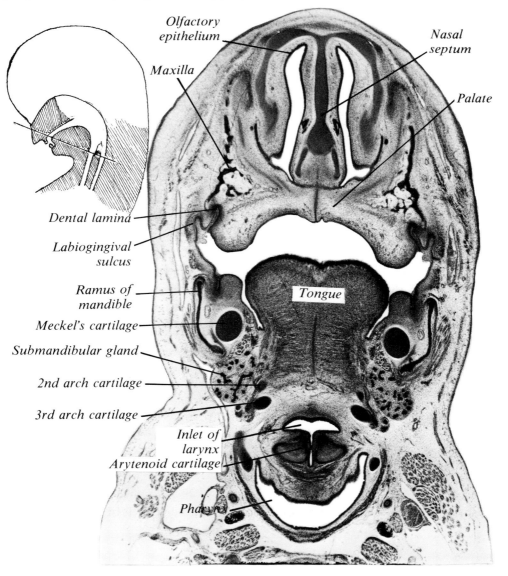

elevation from vertical to horizontal probably depends upon both intrinsic and extrinsic factors. Intrinsic factors include 1) hydration of the glycosaminoglycans within the palatal shelves, and 2) continued growth of the palatal mesenchyme. Extrinsic factors are 1) a gradual flattening of the normal angle between anterior and posterior parts of the cranial base, which may exert a tensile force to assist in elevation, and 2) descent of the tongue within the mouth, sufficient to permit the medial swing of the processes as they assume the horizontal position, sufficient also to provide support for their later medial growth. Since elevation occurs very rapidly—in the rat fetus it can be observed directly and be seen to take less than one second—the intrinsic factor first described (1) is probably the most immediately important.

Fusion of the lateral palatal processes takes place from the incisive foramen backwards, forming the *secondary palate.* The posterior edges of these processes are the last to fuse, creating the *uvula* in the midline of the soft palate. Immediately prior to fusion the epithelial surface along the edge of each lateral palatal process develops a fuzzy coat; a tenuous analogy with the fuzzy coat of small intestinal epithelium suggests that it may contain enzymes concerned in the breakdown of the epithelium along the line of union.

The dorsal part of the frontonasal process lies below the head mesenchyme enclosing the brain. It extends downwards in the midline as the *nasal septum,* which fuses with the upper surface of the palate (Fig. 12-19).

With the completion of the palate, the primitive posterior nares are cut off from the buccal cavity. The *nasal cavity* then extends along the upper surface of the palate on each side of the septum, opening into the pharynx at the *definitive posterior nares,* or *choanae* (Fig. 12-18C).

The cells of the nasal placode form the olfactory epithelium in the upper part of the nasal cavities.

THE TEETH

On the opposed surfaces of upper and lower jaws, paired arclike ectodermal thickenings develop. The first to appear is the *dental lamina* (Fig. 12-21); the second, external to this, deepens to form the *labiogingival groove* and to define the *primitive gum.* At ten points along each jaw the dental lamina proliferates and invades the underlying mesoderm. Each ingrowth is composed of *enamel epithelium.* Its bulbous tip organizes the local mesenchyme, causing it to become a close-packed ball of cells called the *dental papilla.* The enamel epithelium advances to form a cap over the papilla, then encloses it as the bell-shaped *enamel organ.* The outer layer of the bell (*outer enamel epithelium*) is cuboidal epithelium and the inner layer (*inner enamel epithelium*) is columnar; loosely arranged cells form the *enamel pulp* in its core (Fig. 12-22).

The cells of the inner enamel epithelium are known as *ameloblasts.* Under their influence the surface cells of the dental papilla become tall *odontoblasts.* The ameloblasts lay down the dental *enamel.* The odontoblasts form the *dentin* of the tooth. The deeper cells of the dental papilla constitute the *dental pulp* which is invaded by vessels and nerves (Fig. 12-23).

A shell of vascular connective tissue differentiates from the surrounding mesenchyme to enclose the enamel organ and dental papilla. The shell is the *dental sac;* it gives rise to the dental *cement* and to the *periodontal ligament* which attaches the tooth to the bony alveolus (or socket) in which the tooth comes to lie. The dental sac, therefore, completes the formative elements of a tooth, and together with its contents constitutes the *tooth germ.*

As their roots develop, the deciduous teeth erupt through the gums. The incisor teeth are the first to erupt, six months after birth.

The enamel organs of the permanent teeth appear as early as the 12th week after fertilization. On the lingual aspect of each deciduous tooth a bud of enamel epithelium grows from the dental lamina to form a second set of enamel organs. The three permanent molar teeth have no deciduous predecessors; their enamel organs arise by the backward extension of the dental laminae into the posterior wall of the maxilla and into the ramus of the mandible. The further history of the permanent-tooth enamel organs is the same as that of the deciduous set. Eruption commences in the sixth postnatal year, the first permanent molar being the first to erupt.

SALIVARY GLANDS

The three main salivary glands develop as outgrowths from the stomodeal ectoderm during the sixth to eighth weeks of gestation (Fig. 12-21). The acini develop from the duct epithelium during the second half of gestation.

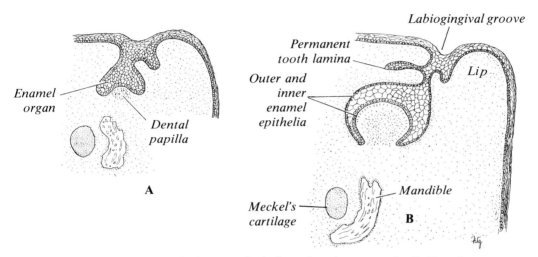

FIG. 12-22. Development of an incisor tooth in the lower jaw: **A,** seven weeks; **B,** 17 weeks.

FIG. 12-23. Development of an incisor tooth (continued): **A,** 24 weeks; **B,** one year after birth.

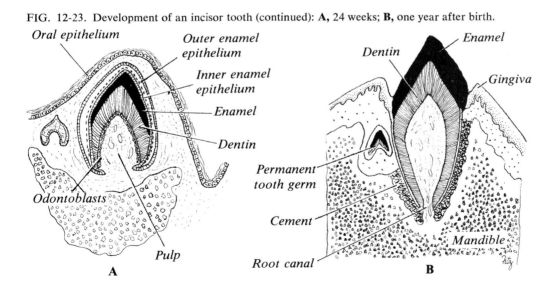

PHARYNGEAL POUCHES AND THYROID GLAND

The pharyngeal (branchial) pouches are the endodermal pockets in the side of the pharynx, between successive pharyngeal arches. The upper four pouches are well defined, the fifth poorly.

The ventral part of the first pouch is obliterated by the developing tongue, while its dorsal part enters the tubotympanic recess (see section "Middle Ear").

TONSIL

The tonsil is first visible as a localized endodermal proliferation in the second pouch, giving rise to the reticular-cell framework of the organ. During the second half of gestation the interstices are invaded by lymphocytes which multiply to form lymph follicles. The *intratonsillar cleft* persists into adult life as a remnant of the second pouch.

THYMUS

The thymus has a bilateral origin from the third pouches. The thymic primordia lose contact with the parent mesoderm and lie on the subjacent fourth aortic arches. They descend on these arches, growing forwards at the same time to meet in the midline. The thymus completes its development in front of the ascending aorta (Fig. 12-24).

Thymocytes, which resemble small lymphocytes, appear in the cortex of the thymus during the ninth week. Experimental work suggests that the stem cells of all the lymphoid cell types originate in the wall of the yolk sac. The stem cells evidently migrate from the yolk sac either to the thymus (to become thymocytes) or to the lymph nodes and bone marrow. Thymocytes proliferate rapidly during fetal life, and interactions between thymus-derived lymphocytes (T cells) and lymphocytes formed in lymph nodes and bone marrow (B cells) take place during the development of normal immunologic processes.

The thymus attains its maximum *relative* size at full term (in relation to body weight). After birth it grows more slowly, and reaches its maximum *absolute* size at puberty.

PARATHYROID GLANDS

The parathyroid glands develop from the third and fourth pouches. The superior parathyroid arises from the *fourth;* it enlarges *in situ,* making contact with the upper pole of the

FIG. 12-24. The thyroid and thymus glands at birth. (From a dissection)

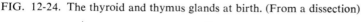
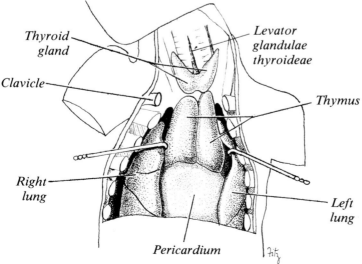

expanding thyroid gland. The inferior parathyroid arises from the *third* pouch, in front of the corresponding thymic lobe. It descends with the thymus, parting company with it near the lower pole of the thyroid. Occasionally, it descends into the thorax with the thymus.

THYROID GLAND

The thyroid gland, although bilobed, probably has but a single origin—from a median proliferation of endoderm just caudal to the mandibular arch (Fig. 12-15). The median thyroid rudiment sinks into the mesoderm overlying the aortic sac. As the aortic sac descends, the thyroid descends in company with the thymus and inferior parathyroid glands. The path taken by the thyroid through the neck is shown for a time by the *thyroglossal duct,* a cord of cells linking the gland to the pharyngeal endoderm. The median rudiment quickly bifurcates to form two lobes connected by an *isthmus.* The *pyramidal lobe,* projecting upwards from the isthmus, or the *levator glandulae thyroideae,* attached to the hyoid bone, may develop to mark the position of the lower part of the thyroglossal duct (Fig. 12-24).

THE EYE

The eye develops from three primordia. An outgrowth from the brain forms the *retina.* An ingrowth of surface (skin) ectoderm forms the *lens.* The local mesoderm gives rise to the *fibrous* and *vascular* coats.

Where it is touched by the optic vesicle, the surface ectoderm thickens to form the *lens placode* (Fig. 12-2). The placode recedes beneath the surface, being converted into the hollow *lens vesicle.* The ectoderm reunites and mesoderm passes between it and the lens vesicle.

As the lens primordium sinks inwards, the optic vesicle becomes a concave *optic cup* to receive it (Fig. 12-25A). Formation of the cup may not be the result of mere pressure by the lens, because the invagination extends along the under surface of the cup and optic stalk to form the *optic fissure.* The lips of the optic fissure fuse during the sixth week of gestation.

The cells of the posterior wall of the lens vesicle elongate to fill its lumen and make contact with the cuboidal cells of the anterior wall. The optic cup gives origin to the *retina.* Its outer wall remains one cell thick throughout life, but its inner wall elaborates the ventricular, intermediate, and marginal zones characteristic of the neural tube from which it originated.

FIG. 12-25. Development of the eye.
A. Diagram of the optic fissure, which is occupied by the hyaloid vessels; the optic stalk is hollow.
B. Infiltration of the optic cup by mesenchyme; the optic fissure has deepened to accommodate the hyaloid vessels, and the cavity of the optic stalk is being obliterated.

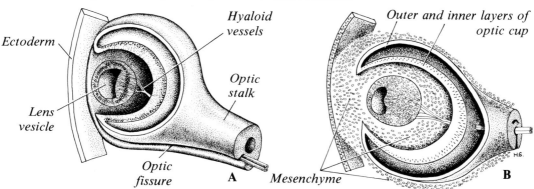

Vascular mesenchyme infiltrates the optic fissure and migrates along it into the optic cup (Fig. 12-25B). In the cup the interstices of the mesenchyme become filled with gelatinous *vitreous humor* (Fig. 12-26B). The *hyaloid vessels* enter the fissure and traverse the vitreous to ramify on the lens (Fig. 12-26A). As the lens matures the distal parts of the hyaloid vessels atrophy. Closure of the optic fissure includes the proximal parts of the vessels in the optic stalk, where they form the *central artery and vein* of the retina. The *hyaloid canal* persists to mark the passage of the vessels through the vitreous.

RETINA AND OPTIC NERVE

The outer epithelial layer of the optic cup is invaded by pigment, to complete the *pigment layer* of the definitive retina. The inner epithelial layer forms the nervous part of the retina, differentiating into photoreceptors, bipolar neurons, and ganglionic neurons. The central processes of the ganglionic neurons form the *nerve fiber layer* of the retina; they converge upon the optic stalk and enter it along the inner wall of the optic fissure, forming the *optic nerve* (Fig. 12-27). The function of the fissure is to provide a direct pathway for the axons of the ganglionic cells. Without it, there would be no exit from the optic cup save at its rim.

Soon after the completion of the lens vesicle a cleft appears in the mesoderm between it and the skin ectoderm. This is the primitive *anterior chamber* of the eye. A tongue of ectoderm extends in front of the lens from the margin of the retina to form the *iris*. For a time the mesoderm stretches across the front of the lens as the *pupillary membrane*. Before birth the part that is unsupported by ectoderm breaks down to define the *pupil*. The interval between the iris and the lens is the *posterior chamber* of the eye. The *sphincter* and *dilator pupillae* muscles develop, probably from the ectoderm, at the free margin of the iris. These and the arrectores pilorum of the skin are the only muscles thought to develop from ectoderm. The *ciliary muscle* arises from the mesoderm near the base of the iris.

The mesoderm forms a fibrous shell around the eye, giving rise to the *substantia propria* of the cornea, the *sclera,* and the *dural sheath* of the optic nerve. Vascular, pigmented mesoderm forms the *choroid coat* of the eyeball, between sclera and retina (Fig. 12-27).

The six extrinsic ocular muscles differentiate outside the sclera, to which they become attached. They are thought to arise from ill-defined *pre-otic myotomes* situated

FIG. 12-26. **A.** Sagittal section of the eye at six weeks. (x50)
B. Section of the optic cup at six and one-half weeks, taken lateral to the plane of the optic fissure. (Cambridge Collection) (x50)

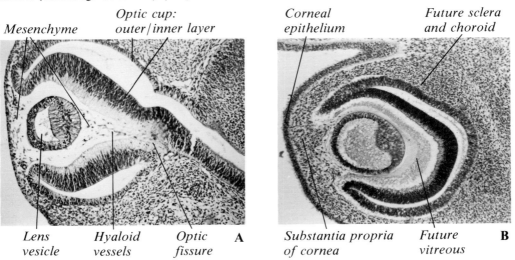

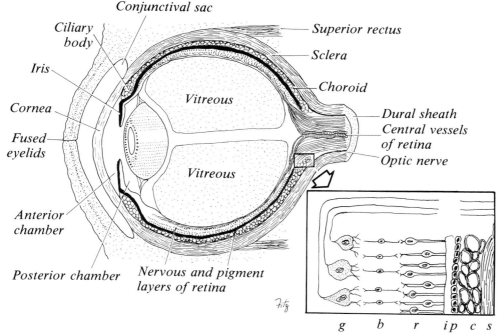

FIG. 12-27. Development of the eye nearing completion, at about 24 weeks. Inset, enlargement of the rectangle at junction of retina with optic nerve. **g,** Ganglion cell layer; **b,** bipolar cell layer; **r,** rod and cone layer; **i,** intraretinal space (cavity of embryonic optic cup); **p,** pigment layer; **c,** choroid; **s,** sclera.

close to the orbit. Their motor nerves—the third, fourth, and sixth cranial—arise in nuclei of the somatic efferent column in the brain stem.

EYELIDS AND LACRIMAL APPARATUS

The eyelids are mesodermal folds, lined with ectoderm, that grow to meet each other in front of the cornea during the second month of gestation. From the third to fifth months the conjunctival sac is sealed by fusion of the apposed epithelial edges of the lids (Fig. 12-27).

The *lacrimal gland* develops from the outer part of the conjunctival sac, in the manner of exocrine glands elsewhere.

A crying newborn infant is not tearful; hence the common belief that the lacrimal gland is nonfunctional at this time. A continuous secretion is, however, present in order to protect the cornea.

THE EAR

INNER EAR

The otic placode appears at the end of the third week of gestation (Fig. 6-14). It recedes beneath the surface to form the *otocyst* (Fig. 12-28A). In doing so it sheds a group of cells beside the hindbrain. These cells constitute the *statoacoustic ganglion*. They assume bipolar form, sending central processes to the vestibular and cochlear nuclei in the myelencephalon, and peripheral processes to the labyrinth and cochlea as these develop.

The *endolymphatic pouch* grows from the otocyst, which then constricts it at its center to form the *vestibular pouch* and the *cochlear pouch* (Fig. 12-28B). The opening of the

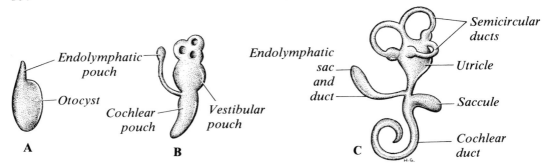

FIG. 12-28. The inner ear: **A,** the otocyst at five weeks; **B,** vestibular and cochlear pouches at six weeks; **C,** further differentiation at seven weeks. (Adapted from Streeter JL: Contrib Embryol Carnegie Inst 7:5, 1918)

endolymphatic pouch shifts to the level of the constriction, and the pouch elongates to become the *endolymphatic duct* and *sac* (Fig. 12-28C).

From the vestibular pouch three platelike expansions give rise to the *semicircular ducts.* The remainder of the pouch persists as the *utricle.* The epithelium lining the pouch forms four vestibular sense organs—the three ampullary *cristae,* and the *macula* of the utricle.

From the cochlear pouch arises the coiled *cochlear duct.* The remainder of this pouch is the future *saccule.* The epithelium of the pouch forms one vestibular sense organ (the macula of the saccule) and the sensory end-organ of hearing (the *organ of Corti*). This completes the *membranous labyrinth,* which is entirely ectodermal in origin.

The *bony labyrinth* results from the ossification of the *otic capsule,* which is a shell of chondrified mesoderm surrounding the membranous labyrinth (Fig. 12-29B). The loose mesenchyme enclosed by the capsule breaks down to produce the *perilymphatic space.*

MIDDLE EAR

During the fourth week of gestation an endodermal diverticulum, the *tubotympanic recess,* grows laterally from the first branchial pouch (Fig. 12-29A). At the same time a corresponding ectodermal diverticulum—the *external acoustic meatus*—grows inwards from the first branchial cleft. The two blind tubes meet below and lateral to the otocyst; the film of mesoderm between them is the primordium of the *tympanic membrane* (eardrum). The outer end of the tubotympanic recess expands to form the *tympanic cavity,* which abuts against the otocyst. The connection with the pharynx persists as the *auditory (eustachian) tube.*

The *ossicles* develop from the dorsal ends of the first and second branchial arches. At first they lie above the tympanic cavity, embedded in loose mesenchyme (Fig. 12-29B), but the cavity enlarges to incorporate them into the middle ear, conferring a lining of respiratory epithelium on them as it does so.

The *tensor tympani* muscle differentiates from the first arch mesoderm in company with the upper part of the malleus, to which it gains attachment. It is supplied by the mandibular nerve. The *stapedius* differentiates from the second arch, together with the stapes; its nerve is the facial.

OUTER EAR

Until the sixth lunar month the external acoutic meatus contains a plug of ectodermal cells, the *meatal plate* (Fig. 12-29B). This plate normally differentiates into the stratified squamous epithelial lining of the meatus.

The *auricle (pinna)* develops from six *aural hillocks*—three located on the first arch and

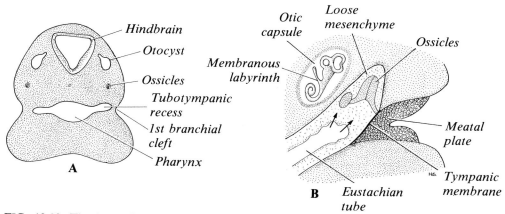

FIG. 12-29. The developing ear: **A,** at four weeks; **B,** eighth week. (Adapted from Pearson AA, Jacobsen AD: The Development of the Ear. Rochester, Minnesota, American Academy of Ophthalmology & Otolaryngology, 1967)

three on the second (Fig. 12-17B). The extent of their respective contributions is unclear. The nerve supply to the skin of the auricle is not a helpful guide, because the mandibular and facial innervation of the outer ear is virtually confined to the external acoustic meatus.

EAR OF THE NEWBORN

The inner ear, tympanic cavity, and ossicles are of adult size at birth. The tympanic antrum, a dorsal extension of the tympanic cavity, is nearly adult in size. On the other hand, mastoid ear cells are absent, as is the mastoid process itself (see section "Skull"). The mastoid process becomes pneumatized as it becomes prominent during the second postnatal year.

The tympanic membrane is nearly horizontal at birth, its upper margin leaning outwards. The lower margin is held in the tympanic ring (see section "Skull"); it is slowly carried laterally with the developing tympanic plate during the first five years of life, and the eardrum becomes more upright. The external acoustic meatus is relatively short at birth, and care must be taken to avoid damage to the eardrum when examining it with a speculum. The meatus elongates with the expansion of the tympanic plate in its floor and the squamous temporal bone in its roof, attaining adult size at about the ninth year.

ABNORMALITIES

THE BRAIN

Anencephaly

Anencephaly, meaning "absence of the brain," is one of the commonest lethal congenital malformations. In various parts of the world its incidence ranges from one to six per 1000 births. Its true frequency is higher than this because many anencephalic embryos are aborted spontaneously.

A full-term anencephalic fetus may be stillborn or may live for a few hours or days. The cerebral hemispheres are absent, giving a characteristic sunken appearance to the head (Fig. 12-30); the diencephalon and midbrain may be absent also. Macerated brain stem tissue is visible through a wide defect in the skin and skull. The pituitary gland is usually present, though small. The body often shows disproportionate enlargement of the shoulder region.

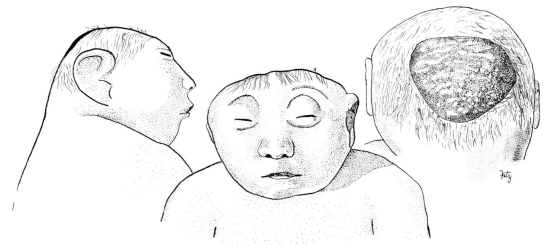

FIG. 12-30. Three views of a full-term anencephalic fetus.

The immediate cause of anencephaly is a growth failure of the telencephalon. The essential nature of the defect is unknown; it may be related to faulty closure of the neural tube.

Hydrocephalus

In hydrocephalus there is an accumulation of cerebrospinal fluid within the ventricular system, or between the brain and dura mater. The enormous head may make normal delivery of the infant impossible. In the absence of surgical treatment, progressive ballooning of the ventricles leads to atrophy of the cerebral cortex. The condition is usually the result of stenosis of the aqueduct of the midbrain, or of the exit foramina of the fourth ventricle. In the *Arnold–Chiari malformation,* hydrocephalus is associated with descent of the medulla oblongata and of the cerebellar vermis through the foramen magnum, and there is an associated spina bifida cystica. According to the commonly held "traction" hypothesis, anchorage of the cord by the spinal defect during development is the primary cause. According to an alternative, "pulsion" hypothesis, the distended brain thrusts the medulla oblongata and cerebellar vermis through the foramen magnum.

FACE AND PALATE

Cleft lip and cleft palate are among the commonest congenital malformations, one or both of these deformities being found about once in every 800 births. The range of deformity varies from isolated unilateral cleft lip to a bilateral cleft lip and cleft palate.

Either genetic or environmental factors may predominate in a particular case. Clefts that are confined to the secondary palate belong to two categories. In one, the influence is primarily genetic; there is a strong family history and the cleft occurs only in female offspring. In the other, the influence is presumed to be environmental as there is no family history or sexual predelection. In cases of cleft lip, with or without a palatal cleft, a mendelian recessive trait operates in conjunction with unknown environmental factors to product the defect.

The histogenesis of the clefts is probably variable. Three mechanisms are possible: 1) The parts may fail to meet because the mesoderm is deficient in amount or is malaligned. 2) Persistence of the ectoderm on the contiguous surfaces may prevent union of the mesoderm. 3) A successful union may be disrupted by traction forces; such a mechanism would account for the connective tissue bands which may traverse a lip cleft.

THE NECK

Branchial Cyst and Fistula

The so-called *branchial* or *lateral cervical cyst* is located close to the anterior margin of the sternomastoid muscle (as a rule) and usually makes its appearance during early adult life. The cyst is usually lined by stratified squamous epithelium surrounded by a shell of lymphoid tissue.

A *branchial fistula* is usually present at birth and may open onto the surface of the neck or into the pharynx. It is lined by columnar epithelium; the pharyngeal opening, when present, is usually in the tonsillar area, i.e., in the region of the second pharyngeal pouch.

The significance of branchial cysts and branchial fistulas is uncertain. A fistula with an internal opening may be derived from one of the pharyngeal pouches. The lymphoid capsule of the cysts suggests either the inclusion of aberrant stratified epithelium within a lymph node during development, or the attraction of lymphoid elements by epithelial cell rests. The source of the epithelium is unknown; its structure suggests an origin from the cervical sinus, but the possibility of aberrant duct cells from the salivary glands cannot be excluded.

Abnormalities of Thyroid Development

Very rarely the thyroid rudiment may fail to descend into the neck. Enlarging *in situ,* it forms a *lingual thyroid gland,* which projects into the oropharynx and may obstruct it.

Persistence of a segment of the thyroglossal duct is more common. It may give rise to cysts or fistulas in the midline of the neck.

THE EYE

Anophthalmia

In anophthalmia, one or both optic vesicles may fail to appear, or may degenerate. The eyeball is absent, but the orbit, eyelids, and extrinsic ocular muscles do develop.

Cyclopia

Cyclopia is a very rare condition characterized by fusion of the optic outgrowths within a single median orbit. The associated malformation of the brain is incompatible with life.

Coloboma of the Iris

In coloboma of the iris a sector of the lower iris is absent, the pupil having the shape of a keyhole. The defect is probably due to faulty closure of the optic fissure. Minor degrees of coloboma are common. Major degrees may be associated with wedge-shaped defects in the ciliary body, choroid, retina, and optic nerve.

Persistent Pupillary Membrane

Partial persistence of the pupillary membrane is not uncommon. Vision is usually unaffected.

Congenital Cataract

A cataract is an opacity of the lens. Congenital cataract is the result of abnormal development of lens fibers. Since the earlier lens fibers are centrally placed and the later fibers are peripheral, the position of the opacity indicates the date of the abnormal development. The condition usually results from maternal infection by the rubella virus, but it may be genetic in origin.

Persistence of Hyaloid Vessels

Remnants of the hyaloid vessels are commonly found on clinical examination of the posterior chamber of the eye. Rarely the vessels are large and maintain the embryonic connective tissue behind the lens, with severe obstruction of vision.

THE EAR

Congenital Deafness

In congenital deafness it is usually the child's failure to develop the faculty of speech that is first noticed. The fault may lie in the sound-conducting pathway (outer and middle ear) or in the sound-perception mechanism (cochlea and its nerve connections). The latter is called *nerve deafness,* and is untreatable. In about one-third of all cases of congenital deafness a hereditary trait is manifested; about one-fifth of the cases are the result of maternal rubella.

Treacher-Collins Syndrome

In the *Treacher–Collins syndrome,* faults in the sound-conducting pathway (meatal atresia, ossicular ankylosis, etc.) result from incomplete mandibular arch development on one or both sides. The mandible and maxilla are reduced in size, so that the distance from external acoustic meatus to the nostril is abnormally short.

SUGGESTED READING

Coulombre AJ: Regulation of ocular morphogenesis. Invest Ophthalmol 8:25–31, 1969

Cowan WM: Neuronal death as a regulation mechanism in the control of cell numbers in the central nervous system. In Rockstein M, Sussman ML (eds): Development and Aging in the Nervous System. New York, Academic Press, 1973, pp 19–42

Davies J: Embryology of the Head and Neck in Relation to the Practice of Otolaryngology. Rochester Minnesota, American Academy of Ophthalmology & Otolaryngology,1965

Dobbing J: Later development of the brain and its vulnerability. In Davis JA, Dobbing J (eds): Scientific Foundations of Pediatrics. London, Heinemann, 1975, pp 565–576

Jacobson M: Histogenesis and morphogenesis of the nervous system. In Jacobson M (ed): Developmental Neurobiology. New York, Holt, Rinehart & Winston, 1970, pp 1–64

Lemire RJ: Embryology of the central nervous system. In David JA, Dobbing J (eds): Scientific Foundations of Pediatrics. London, Heinemann, 1975, pp 547–564

Luke DA: Development of the secondary palate in man. Acta Anat (Basel) 94:596–608, 1976

Muir IFK: Cleft lip and palate—general. Br Med J 3:107–108, 1974

Pearson AA, Jacobson AD: The Development of the Ear. Rochester Minnesota, American Academy of Ophthalmology & Otolaryngology, 1967

Slavin HC, Baretta LA: Developmental Aspects of Oral Biology. New York, Academic Press, 1972

Shepard TH: Development of the human fetal thyroid. Gen Comp Endocrinol 10:174–181, 1968

West CD, Kemper TL: The effect of a low protein diet on the anatomical development of the rat brain. Brain Res 107:221–237, 1976

Windle WF: Central nervous system. In Windle WF (ed): Physiology of the Fetus. Springfield, Ill, C C Thomas, 1971, pp 66–76

I went a thousand miles since they were wed,
from a tiny lowly painprick
to a bursting water bubble
with my heels above my head,
a running, standing, sitting, lying leap
from a double,
to a single bed

M. J. T. FitzGerald

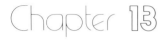

full term

In Chapter 4 it was noted that the placenta arises from the interplay between the chorion frondosum and the decidua basalis. It consists of three parts: 1) the tertiary villi, 2) the superficial part of the decidua basalis, and 3) the intervillous space.

During the middle trimester the placenta develops prodigiously, but the original relationships between fetal and maternal components are maintained. The tertiary villi grow in treelike fashion, developing more and more sideshoots and terminal buds. The growing tips display knoblike thickenings of syncytiotrophoblast which often show clumps of nuclei known as *syncytial knots*. Fresh syncytium is continuously recruited from the cytotrophoblast, which diminishes in amount as pregnancy advances. Progressive erosion of maternal vessels accompanies enlargement of the intervillous space. The maternal capillaries in the decidua basalis are engulfed by the trophoblast, and the spiral arteries and uterine veins are tapped. The decidua is not penetrated beyond the superficial part of the spongy layer. *Placental septa* are narrow ridges of decidua that project into the intervillous space. The septa are more or less cup-shaped, and are interconnected.

During parturition the placenta separates from the decidua along a plane within the spongy layer. The remainder of the spongy layer is also shed, and this and the compact layers regenerate from the intact basal layer in the same manner as in the menstrual cycle.

As the villous stems thicken to become trunks, the umbilical vessels enlarge and the arteries acquire muscle coats. Capillary buds extend into each new subdivision of the chorionic tree. The chorionic investment of the fetal vessels is glovelike.

THE FULL-TERM PLACENTA

POSITION

The most common placental site is the posterior wall of the uterus, near the fundus. Less common sites are the anterior wall (where the placenta may be felt by careful abdominal palpation) and the fundus itself. With repeated pregnancies there is a tendency for the blastocyst to drop to a lower level in the uterus before implantation, and there is a corresponding tendency for the placenta to extend into the *lower segment* of the uterus (the part of the corpus uteri that thins to permit passage of the fetus during parturition), a condition known as *placenta praevia* (*praevia*, in the way).

STRUCTURE

The chorion frondosum, of which the placenta is mainly composed, is continuous with the chorion laeve on all sides. The amniotic sac fills the entire uterine cavity and the amnion presses against the inner, *fetal surface* of the placenta. The outer, *maternal surface* is incorporated into the decidua basalis.

When the freshly delivered placenta is examined, its fetal surface is seen to be smooth and shiny. It is covered by the amnion, which is adherent around the placental margin and invests the umbilical cord. Through the amnion can be seen the umbilical vessels as they fan out before entering the placental substance (Fig. 13-1A).

The umbilical cord is 30–60 cm in length. It is composed of extraembryonic mesenchyme embedded in a mucoid matrix called *Wharton's jelly*. Within the cord are the two umbilical arteries, pursuing a spiral course around the single (left) umbilical vein. The allantois (Fig. 13-2) persists for a variable period within the fetal end of the cord before undergoing atrophy.

The maternal surface of the placenta is rough (Fig. 13-1B). It is divided into 15–20 irregular islands called *maternal cotyledons*. On the surface is a film of decidua sheared from the uterine wall during separation of the placenta. The grooves between them are created by the placental septa.

Dissection of the placenta shows that the thick sheet of chorion—the *chorionic plate*—gives attachment to about 200 chorionic trees, known as *fetal cotyledons,* which project towards the decidua basalis. The decidua basalis, together with the cytotrophoblastic shell on its fetal surface, is called the *basal plate* (Fig. 13-3).

The smallest fetal cotyledons form groups of terminal villi near the chorionic plate. The largest are derived from the enchoring villi of early pregnancy; their anchorage extends from the chorionic plate to the basal plate. Their side branches give rise to a profusion of terminal villi (Fig. 13-3).

FIG. 13-1. Full-term placenta: **A**, fetal surface; **B**, maternal surface.

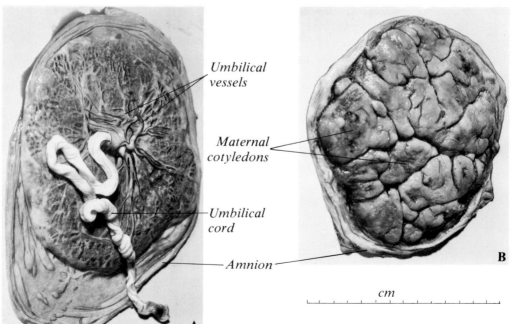

Umbilical vessels

Maternal cotyledons

Umbilical cord

Amnion

cm

A

B

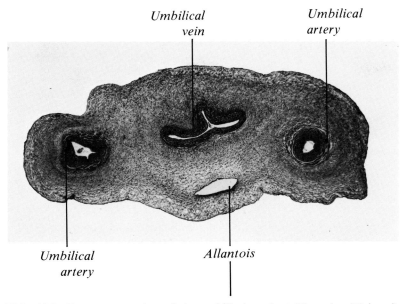

FIG. 13-2. Transverse section of the umbilical cord at 15 weeks. (University of Washington Collection) (x15)

FIG. 13-3. Diagram of portion of the mature placenta. Only one villous tree is represented. NOTE: The intervillous space is normally filled with maternal blood; the **arrows** indicate its direction of flow.

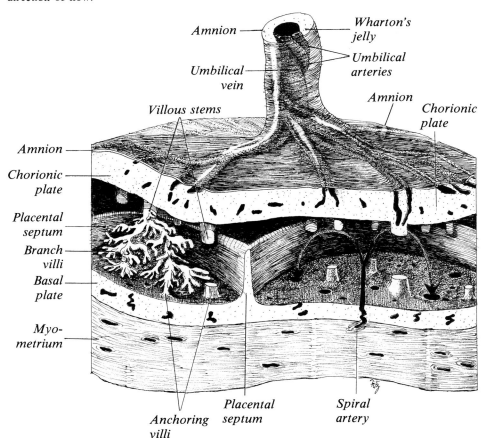

FETAL VESSELS

The two umbilical arteries are highly muscular (Fig. 13-2). They are much smaller than the umbilical vein. They usually anastomose with one another close to the placenta; then they branch dichotomously, the placental territory of each being proportionate to its size. The tributaries of the umbilical vein accompany the arteries.

The large vessels ramify on the fetal surface of the chorionic plate. Their branches sink into its substance to enter the villi. Within the villous stems and their subdivisions, the arteries and veins differ in their arrangement. The arteries divide repeatedly so that several run side by side (Fig. 13-4). Entering the villous branches, they give rise to a profuse paravascular capillary network. The meshes of the network are mainly in line with the parent vessels. At intervals the capillaries drain into adjacent veins.

The branch villi float in the intervillous space. Some are united by syncytial bridges, or by deposits of fibrinoid substance, but their circulation is always independent. Each contains a wide capillary loop that follows the irregular contour of the villus. Its arterial end is fed by a branch of the paravascular capillary plexus; its venous end is linked by a short venule to the nearest tributary vein.

The paravascular capillary network has a dual function. First, by greatly increasing the vascular bed of the branch villi, it slows the flow of blood so that the circulation time through the terminal villous loops is increased and more complete physiologic exchange with the maternal blood is effected. The early division of the arteries to form leashes of parallel vessels (from which the paravascular plexus is derived) is an additional mechanism for reducing the rate of flow. The frequent direct communications between the paravascular capillaries and the adjacent veins provide arteriovenous shunts by which the terminal villous bed may be bypassed. The arrangement may be regarded as a device to prevent overloading of terminal capillary loops.

FIG. 13-4. Component parts of the placenta.

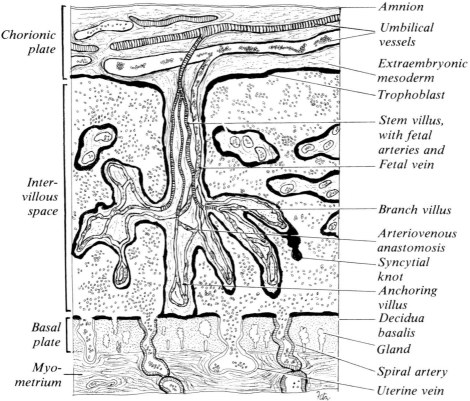

MATERNAL VESSELS

Some 200 spiral arteries open, through short straight segments, into the intervillous space. About 500 ml of maternal blood passes through the intervillous space each minute. The movement of the intervillous blood has not been observed in humans. In monkeys the arterial blood spurts into the intervillous space, reaching the chorionic plate before being dispersed. It returns more slowly, percolating through the villous sponge on its way to the venous exits. Gentle rhythmic contractions of the human uterus (known as *Braxton–Hicks contractions*) are thought to assist in emptying the intervillous space. The anchoring villi contain smooth muscle which, by drawing the chorionic plate towards the basal plate, may prevent the formation of stagnant loculi of maternal blood.

THE PLACENTAL MEMBRANE

The fetal and maternal circulations become more intimately related in later pregnancy. The fetal capillaries widen and come closer to the surface of the terminal villi. The cytotrophoblast cells are flatter and no longer form a continuous lining. The syncytium is thinner also. The *placental membrane,* or *placental barrier,* between fetal and maternal circulations, comprises 1) the fetal capillary endothelium, 2) a thin layer of collagen fibers, 3) the basement membrane of the villus, and 4) a film of syncytiotrophoblast (Fig. 13-5). *The placental barrier is therefore entirely fetal in origin.*

Direct communication between the fetal and maternal blood streams has not been demonstrated histologically. However, in about 45% of pregnant women, films of the peripheral blood reveal fetal erythrocytes. Intermittent discharge of fetal cells into the maternal blood may quite possibly be a normal event. The matter has an important bearing on the development of *Rhesus incompatibility.* If a Rhesus-negative woman bears a child by a Rhesus-positive man, the fetus may be Rhesus-positive. Fetal erythrocytes may cross the placental barrier and stimulate the production of antibodies. The antibodies, returning to the fetus, will react with the fetal Rhesus antigens, causing intravascular hemolysis. The condition is known as *hemolytic disease of the newborn* (erythroblastosis fetalis); it does not usually develop in the first offspring of a Rhesus-negative mother and Rhesus-positive father, but in subsequent ones it is common.

PHYSIOLOGY OF THE PLACENTA

In addition to providing an anatomic partition between fetal and maternal circulations, the placenta has four functions: 1) to act as a fetal *lung* for the purpose of respiratory exchange;

FIG. 13-5. The placental membrane.

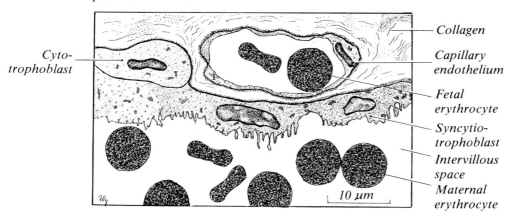

Cytotrophoblast — Collagen — Capillary endothelium — Fetal erythrocyte — Syncytiotrophoblast — Intervillous space — Maternal erythrocyte

10 µm

2) to act as an *intestine* in providing nutriments—amino acids, sugars, lipids, minerals, and vitamins; 3) to act as a *kidney* for the elimination of the end products of fetal metabolism; and 4) to produce *hormones* necessary for the maintenance of pregnancy.

TRANSFER MECHANISMS

Diffusion

The placenta acts as a semipermeable membrane to permit the free diffusion, in both directions, of solutes of low molecular weight. Water and electrolytes pass rapidly across the membrane, equilibrium being attained in seconds. The rate of sodium transfer from mother to fetus rises steeply up to the eighth month of gestation; presumably the increasing rate of sodium transfer is related to the concomitant thinning of the placental barrier. Oxygen does not attain equilibrium because of rapid utilization by the fetus. The mean oxygen saturation of intervillous blood is about 70%; that of umbilical venous blood is about 65%. Carbon dioxide diffuses more rapidly than oxygen. Minerals (*e.g.,* calcium, iron, phosphorus) are also rapid, as are the molecules of the volatile anesthetics used in the management of labor. The large molecules of the steroid and protein hormones produced by the maternal endocrine glands diffuse very slowly to the fetus.

Active Transport

Molecules required for the nutrition of growing organs are transferred by active transport. Carrier molecules are believed to shuttle back and forth within the placental membrane, taking the selected substances from the maternal to the fetal surface. This mechanism accounts (in part) for the passage of glucose from mother to fetus. Because of rapid utilization, the glucose level of fetal blood is lower than that of maternal blood. Amino acids, on the other hand, are more concentrated in fetal blood, so that the carrier system must operate against the concentration gradient. Lipids are partially catabolized at the maternal surface before being transferred actively to the fetus.

Pinocytosis and Reverse Pinocytosis

Pinocytotic activity at the free surface of the syncytium may be a mechanism for the incorporation of very large molecules into the placental membrane. Cytoplasmic vesicles formed by pinocytosis appear to be discharged into the fetal villi by reverse pinocytosis. Gamma globulins may be transmitted in this way; certainly the child acquires a passive immunity to viral infections, *e.g.,* measles, whooping cough, acquired by the mother in earlier life. Viruses themselves can cross the placenta, as witness the fetal injury that may follow maternal infection by the virus of German measles. Bacteria, however, cannot utilize the normal transport mechanisms; fetal bacterial disease is always secondary to infection of the placental villi.

SYNTHETIC ACTIVITY

Chorionic gonadotropin is a glycoprotein synthesized by the trophoblast. Its function is to maintain the corpus luteum until the placenta is itself capable of producing estrogen and progesterone. During implantation it diffuses freely into the maternal blood within the trophoblastic lacunae. During the third week after implantation commences (during the second week after the first missed menstruation) the hormone is detectable in the maternal blood and urine. This finding is the basis of several pregnancy tests. Production of chorionic gonadotropin rises to a peak during the third month; thereafter, it declines to a low level.

From the fourth week onwards, the placenta forms estrogen and progesterone in increasing amounts. By the end of the fifth week their concentration is usually sufficient to maintain pregnancy. Removal of the ovary that contains the corpus luteum of pregnancy, therefore, leads to placental degeneration (and death of the embryo) if carried out before the fifth week; if carried out later, the procedure is usually without ill effect.

The fetal liver begins to function in the third month. Until then the placenta is the *fetal glycogen reserve*. The early trophoblast is also rich in ribosomes, indicating active protein synthesis; and it is probable that *fetal plasma proteins* are synthesized here until the liver assumes this function.

AMNIOTIC FLUID

The normal volume of amniotic fluid at the end of pregnancy (*full term*) ranges from 500 to 2,000 ml. Prior to the 15th week of pregnancy its principal source is the lining epithelium of the amniotic sac. Later the fetal kidneys are the main source. The composition of amniotic fluid resembles that of dilute urine, containing small amounts of urea, uric acid, nonprotein nitrogen, and sodium chloride.

The amniotic fluid *circulates* as follows: it is swallowed by the fetus, absorbed from the alimentary tract into the blood stream, excreted by the fetal kidneys, and returned by the urinary tract to the amniotic sac. Congenital malformations may interfere with this circulation. In bilateral renal agensis, for example, fluid is absent from the amnotic sac at full term. In congenital atresia of the duodenum the amount of fluid is excessive—presumably because of interference with absorption.

With the onset of labor, uterine contractions force a cone of amnion, with its investing chorion laeve, into the cervical canal, which responds by a slow dilatation. The amniotic fluid then bursts through the membranes and a variable amount escapes through the vagina ("rupture of the membranes," "escape of the waters") before the cervix is plugged for a time by the descending fetal head.

FETAL CIRCULATION

The fetal circulation is illustrated in Figure 13-6, to which the numbers in parentheses in the following four paragraphs refer.

The umbilical vein (**1**) delivers blood at about 65% oxygen saturation to the fetus. Upon reaching the liver, almost all the blood passes in the ductus venosus to the stem of the inferior vena cava. A small amount is diverted into the venae advehentes of the portal vein; it circulates through the liver substance, returning to the inferior vena cava in the venae revehentes and hepatic veins. A significant amount of reduced blood is added from the inferior vena cava (**2**), which returns blood to the heart from the abdomen, pelvis, and lower limbs.

The right atrium of the heart (**3**) has two principal entrances—the caval orifices—and two exits—the foramen ovale and the right atrioventricular orifice. The four openings are so disposed that blood entering by the inferior vena cava is directed through the foramen ovale (**4**) to the left atrium, while that entering by the superior vena cava finds its way through the atrioventricular orifice to the right ventricle. In this way the two channels of blood form the very remarkable *crossing streams* within the right atrium. The streams are not completely separate, however. The extent to which they mingle in humans is uncertain, but comparative observations suggest that up to one-quarter of the inferior caval blood is deflected into the right ventricle.

From the left atrium (**5**) the blood, at about 60% saturation, passes to the left ventricle (**6**) and thence to the ascending aorta (**7**). The left ventricular blood is distributed to the

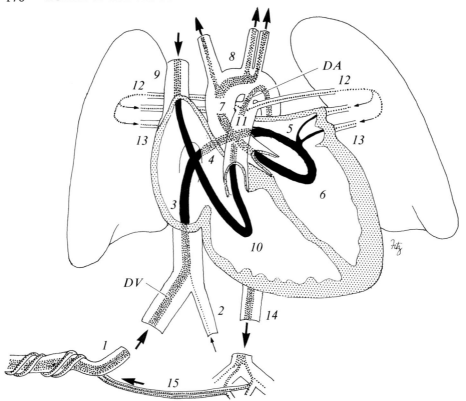

FIG. 13-6. Diagram of the fetal circulation. DA, ductus arteriosus; DV, ductus venosus.

head, neck, and upper limbs through the three great vessels (**8**) arising from the aortic arch. It returns by the jugular and subclavian veins, which convey it to the superior vena cava (**9**). Having passed through the right atrium and ventricle (**10**) it is pumped into the pulmonary trunk (**11**). Of the three available outlets from the pulmonary trunk, the ductus arteriosus is wide and lies in the axis of flow of the ventricular blood; the pulmonary arteries (**12**) are small and are at an angle to the axis of flow. Accordingly, the bulk of the blood enters the aorta through the ductus; a small residuum runs through the pulmonary vascular bed, to be returned to the left atrium by way of the pulmonary veins (**13**).

The ductus arteriosus is attached to the distal extremity of the aortic arch. The arch proper being filled with left ventricular blood, the input from the ductus is deflected into the descending aorta (**14**). Most of this blood is returned to the placenta in the umibilical arteries (**15**); the remainder is distributed to the trunk and lower extremities.

CIRCULATORY CHANGES AT BIRTH

Two events following birth have a dramatic effect on the circulation. 1) Blood flow ceases in the umbilical vessels following either their spontaneous constriction or clamping by the obstetrician's forceps. Pressure in the ductus venosus drops to zero, causing a sharp fall of pressure in the right atrium. 2) With the first expansion of the chest, the pulmonary vascular bed opens up and blood is diverted to the lungs. The raised oxygen tension in the blood produced by pulmonary ventilation has a curious double effect; it relaxes the smooth muscle of the pulmonary arteries, promoting the vascular perfusion of the lungs, and it causes the smooth muscle cells of the ductus arteriosus to contract thereby occluding its lumen.

The increased pulmonary flow returns to the left atrium, raising the blood pressure there. The combined effect of lower right atrial pressure and elevated left atrial pressure ensures that the flaplike septum primum is apposed to the septum secundum, thereby occluding the foramen ovale. The left atrial blood is deflected to the left ventricle and thence to the aorta. With the loss of input to the aorta from the ductus arteriosus, the left ventricular output becomes responsible for perfusion of the entire systemic arterial tree.

The wall of the ductus venosus is slowly replaced by fibrous tissue. Its remnants in the adult are the *ligamentum teres,* in the free edge of the falciform ligament, and the *ligamentum venosum,* which connects the portal vein to the stem of the inferior vena cava. Curiously, the lumens of both ligaments remain patent throughout life.

In the ductus arteriosus a deposit of fibrin on its intimal surface is slowly invaded by fibroblasts. The swollen muscle cells in the wall of the ductus are also replaced by fibrous tissue and the adult remnant of the ductus is the *ligamentum arteriosum,* which attaches the commencement of the left pulmonary artery to the under aspect of the aortic arch.

Around the rim of the foramen ovale, fibrinous adhesions develop within a few days of birth between the septum primum and septum secundum. The two septa adhere, and permanent bonding is brought about by invading fibroblasts.

CIRCULATION AFTER BIRTH

Circulation after birth is illustrated in Figure 13-7, to which the numbers in parentheses in the following paragraph refer.

From the inferior vena cava (**1**) and superior vena cava (**2**) venous blood enters the right atrium (**3**). The entire blood flow passes to the right ventricle (**4**), from which it is ejected through the pulmonary trunk (**5**) into the pulmonary arteries (**6**). Oxygenated

FIG. 13-7. Diagram of the circulation after birth. LA, ligamentum arteriosum; LV, ligamentum venosum.

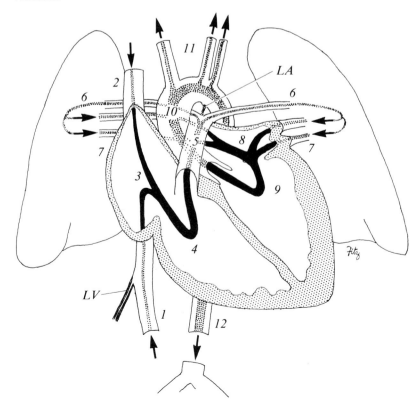

blood returns from the lungs by the four pulmonary veins (**7**) to the left atrium (**8**), which transmits it to the left ventricle (**9**). Finally, left ventricular contraction fills the ascending aorta (**10**) and the aortic arch, from which the great arteries of the head, neck, and upper limbs are given off (**11**). The remainder of the arterial blood is distributed by the descending aorta (**12**) to the trunk and lower limbs.

ABNORMALITIES

PLACENTA

Occasionally a material cotyledon is separated from the main mass to which it is attached by a vascular stalk. This *succenturiate, i.e.,* accessory, *lobe* may remain in the uterus after delivery and cause severe postpartum hemorrhage.

The attachment of the umbilical cord is usually eccentric. Less commonly it is central or marginal. Rarely the umbilical vessels ramify on the chorion laeve before entering the placenta, a condition called *velamentous insertion of the cord.*

Rarely the chorionic villi penetrate the decidua basalis completely and enter the myometrium, a condition called *placenta increta.* In the most advanced form (*placenta percreta*) the villi broach the visceral peritoneum investing the uterus. Penetration of the myometrium by the chorion may be due to faulty development of the decidual reaction at the time of implantation.

Three degrees of placenta praevia are recognized: 1) central, where the placenta straddles the internal os; 2) lateral, where the lower edge reaches the internal os; and 3) marginal, where the lower edge reaches only to the lower uterine segment. In first pregnancies the incidence of placenta praevia is about 0.2%; in fifth, about 5%. The condition is dangerous both to mother and fetus because the placenta separates prematurely during parturition, giving rise to antepartum hemorrhage from torn blood vessels.

AMNIOTIC FLUID

Hydramnios is a common abnormality (one in 200 pregnancies) in which there is a clinically demonstrable excess of amniotic fluid. Anencephaly is an associated finding in about one-fifth of cases. In terms of the circulation of the amniotic fluid, the responsible feature in the anencephalic may be absence of the neurohypophysis; for polyuria, *i.e.,* greatly increased output of dilute urine, always results from deficiency of the antidiuretic hormone produced by the neurohypophysis. The relationship of congenital duodenal atresia to hydramnios has been referred to.

Oligohydramnios (*oligoamnios*) is the rare condition in which the volume of amniotic fluid is less than 500 ml. Whenever the fluid is completely absent, renal agenesis should be suspected.

Oligohydramnios has an established linkage with *postural deformities* of the newborn. Postural deformities are distinguishable from malformations in that they occur after the completion of morphogenesis; their incidence before the 20th week is very low (about 0.1% of abortuses) and after the 28th week may be as high as 2%. This late onset is due to *molding* of the rapidly growing fetus by the uterus. Compression of the fetus is more likely if the amount of amniotic fluid is less than normal. An extreme instance is *Potter's facies,* in which renal malformation (with little or no amniotic fluid) is associated with compression deformity of the face and ears. Postural deformities of the feet, congenital dislocation of the hip, and congenital postural scoliosis are other examples.

Amniotic fluid contains a suspension of cells derived from the fetal skin, respiratory and alimentary tracts, and from the amniotic epithelium. In the procedure known as *amniocen-*

tesis, a needle is inserted into the amniotic sac through the lower abdominal wall. Amniotic fluid is withdrawn, centrifuged, and the cells are cultured and then karyotyped. The procedure is feasible from the 15th week of gestation onwards; it is used when the case history indicates a likelihood of fetal chromosomal disorder.

The concentration of *α-fetoprotein* in amniotic fluid is markedly elevated in the presence of open neural tube defects (myelocele, anencephaly).

UMBILICAL CORD

The umbilical vein commonly forms small loops that are covered with Wharton's jelly; the resultant nodes, or *false knots,* are of no significance. *True knots* are rare; they may develop at any time by the passage of the fetus through a looped cord. Fetal movements may draw the knot tight and cause fetal death from asphyxia.

An unduly long umbilical cord may be coiled around the fetal neck or trunk, leading to the risk of death from asphyxia. A very short cord is rare, but it is also dangerous; during delivery of the fetus it may pull on the placenta, causing it to separate prematurely. Such a cord has been known to turn the uterus inside out (*eversion* of the uterus) by exerting traction on the fundus.

SUGGESTED READING

Bøe F: Vascular morphology of the human placenta. Cold Spring Harbor Symp Quant Biol 19:29–35, 1954

Boyd JD, Hamilton WJ: The Human Placenta. Cambridge, Heffer, 1970

Burchell RC: Arterial blood flow into the human intervillous space. Am J Obstet Gynecol 98:303–311, 1967

Davies GS: The foetal circulation. In Foetal and Neonatal Physiology. Chicago, Year Book Medical, 1968, pp 91–105

Dunn P: Congenital postural deformities: further perinatal associations. Proc R Soc Med 67:32–36, 1974

Ramsey EM, Martin CB, Donner MW: Fetal and maternal placental circulations. Fertil Steril 98:419–423, 1967

glossary

glossary of embryologic terms

ACROSOME REACTION Liberation of acrosomal contents during penetration of the corona radiata

AGENESIS Failure of development

ALAR PLATE Dorsal part of neural tube

ALLANTOIS Endodermal diverticulum extending from yolk sac into body stalk

AMELIA Absence of the limbs

AMNION Flat-celled membrane secreted by the trophoblast, attached to the margin of the ectoderm

AMNIOTIC SAC Vesicle enclosed by amnion and ectoderm

ANAL MEMBRANE Posterior division of cloacal membrane

ANAL PIT Depression external to anal membrane

ANCHORING VILLUS Villus attached to decidua basalis

ANENCEPHALY Absence of the forebrain

ANGIOBLAST Precursor of capillary endothelium

ANTRUM, FOLLICULAR Cavity of graafian follicle, contains liquor folliculi

AORTIC SAC Expanded distal end of truncus arteriosus

APICAL ECTODERMAL RIDGE Ectodermal thickening at tip of limb bud

ATHELIA Absence of nipple

ATRESIA Failure of development

AZOOSPERMIA Absence of live sperm in the semen

BASAL PLATE Ventral part of neural tube

BILAMINAR EMBRYONIC DISK Apposed ectoderm and endoderm before appearance of mesoderm

BLASTOCYST Sphere of cells comprising trophoblast and embryoblast

BLASTOMERES The cells produced by cleavage of the zygote, including those of the morula

BLOOD ISLANDS Islands of hemopoiesis on the surface of the yolk sac

BODY STALK Extraembryonic mesoderm connecting embryo to chorion

BRAIN PLATE Expanded rostral part of neural plate

BRANCH VILLUS Branch of stem villus, occupies intervillous space

BRANCHIAL ARCHES Mesodermal bars in sides and floor of pharynx

BRANCHIAL GROOVES (CLEFTS) Ectodermal depressions between successive branchial arches

BRANCHIAL POUCHES Endodermal depressions between successive branchial arches

BUCCOPHARYNGEAL MEMBRANE See Oral membrane

BUD First rudiment, or primordium

CAPACITATION Conferring of ability of sperm to fertilize by passage through the uterus

CARDIOGENIC CRESCENT Mesoderm giving rise to heart tubes

CAUDAL MESODERM The mesoderm caudal to, and beside, the cloacal membrane

CHORION The trophoblast together with the underlying extraembryonic mesoderm

CHORION FRONDOSUM The chorion penetrating the decidua basalis

CHORION LAEVE "Smooth" chorion under decidua capsularis

CHORIONIC PLATE The chorion on the fetal surface of the mature placenta; contains the main branches of the umbilical vessels

183

CHORIONIC VESICLE (SAC) The vesicle bounded by the chorion and containing the embryo

CLEAVAGE The phase of repeated cell division that transforms the zygote into a morula

CLOACA Hindgut caudal to the allantois

CLOACAL MEMBRANE Area of adhesion of ectoderm and endoderm caudal to the primitive streak

COELOM *See* Embryonic coelom; Extraembryonic coelom

COMPETENCE Ability of cells to respond to organizers

CONCEPTUS The product of conception—embryo and membranes

CONGENITAL MALFORMATION Abnormality present at birth

CORONA RADIATA Radially arranged granulosa cells surrounding secondary oocyte after ovulation

CORPUS ALBICANS Scarred remnant of corpus luteum

CORPUS LUTEUM Endocrine gland derived from the ruptured graafian follicle

CORTICAL REACTION Reaction of cortex of ovum to penetration by spermatozoon

COTYLEDONS *See* Fetal cotyledons; Maternal cotyledons

CYTOTROPHOBLAST Cellular layer of trophoblast

CYTOTROPHOBLASTIC SHELL Shell of cytotrophoblast surrounding the chorionic vesicle; anchoring villi are attached to it

DECIDUA The endometrium of pregnancy

DECIDUA BASALIS Decidua to which chorion frondosum is attached

DECIDUA CAPSULARIS Decidua enclosing chorionic vesicle

DECIDUA PARIETALIS Decidua not invaded by chorion

DENTAL LAMINA Ectodermal precursor of enamel organ

DENTAL SAC Mesenchyme surrounding enamel organ

DERMATOME Subdivision of the somite; forms dermis of skin

DERMOMYOTOME Temporary union of dermatome and myotome

DIENCEPHALON The median part of the forebrain comprising epithalamus, thalamus, and hypothalamus

DIFFERENTIATION Structural change within a cell (or cell group) leading to the production of new cell types

DIGITAL RAYS Mesenchymal precursors of metacarpal (metatarsal) tissues and of the digits

DUCTUS ARTERIOSUS Channel connecting left pulmonary artery to aortic arch

DUCTUS VENOSUS Channel connecting (left) umbilical vein to inferior vena cava

ECTODERM Germ layer that gives rise to the nervous system and the epidermis of the skin

ECTOPIA Abnormal location of an organ or tissue

ECTROMELIA Absence of an individual limb

EMBRYO The organism in the period from the completion of implantation until the end of the eighth week of gestation

EMBRYOLOGY The study of prenatal development

EMBRYONIC (INTRAEMBRYONIC) COELOM The serous cavity formed within the embryo; forms pericardial, pleural, and peritoneal cavities

EMBRYONIC DISK Disk-shaped early embryo composed of two (later, three) germ layers

EMBRYONIC (INTRAEMBRYONIC) MESODERM The mesoderm formed from the primitive streak

EMBRYONIC PHARYNX *See* Pharynx

ENAMEL ORGAN Ectodermal precursor of tooth enamel; composed of outer and inner enamel epithelium and enamel pulp

ENDODERM The germ layer that forms the epithelium of the embryonic gut and its derivatives

EPIMERE Dorsal subdivision of the myotome

EXTRAEMBRYONIC COELOM The cavity surrounding the embryo, within the chorionic vesicle

EXTRAEMBRYONIC MESODERM Mesoderm delaminated from inner surface of trophoblast; forms the connective tissue elements of the chorion, including the vessels of the placenta and umbilical cord

FEMALE PRONUCLEUS Nucleus of ovum at fertilization

FETAL COTYLEDONS Treelike colonies formed by branching of stem villi. The term "cotyledon" used alone implies a maternal (placental) cotyledon

FETAL MEMBRANES Amnion, chorion, yolk sac remnant, and allantois

FETUS The organism in the period from the beginning of the eighth week of gestation until full term

FIBRINOID SUBSTANCE Fibrinous material on the maternal surface of the trophoblast

FLEXION Formation of the head, tail, and lateral body folds

FOREGUT (EMBRYONIC) The gut extending from the oral membrane to the level of the vitelline duct; forms definitive pharynx, esophagus, and definitive foregut (from gastroesophageal junction to point of entry of bile duct)

GAMETE The mature male or female sex cell

GAMETOGENESIS Development of the male and female gametes

GENITAL TUBERCLE Primordium of the phallus

GERM CELLS The gametes

GERM LAYERS The ectoderm, embryonic mesoderm, and endoderm

GERM PLASM The line of cells that gives rise to a gamete

GRAAFIAN FOLLICLE Ovarian follicle after appearance of the antrum

GUBERNACULUM In males, the fibrous anchor of the testis; in females, the procursor of the round ligament of the uterus and ligament of the ovary

HEAD FOLD The rostral body fold

HEAD MESENCHYME Diffuse mesodermal investment of the developing brain; forms the skull and the upper part of the face

HEPATIC BUD Endodermal primordium of liver and biliary tract

HINDGUT (EMBRYONIC) The gut extending from vitelline duct to cloacal membrane

HISTOGENESIS Development of a tissue

HYOID ARCH Second branchial arch

HYPOMERE Ventral subdivision of the myotome

IMPLANTATION Embedding of the fertilized ovum in the endometrium

INDUCTION Action of one cell group upon another to influence its development

INGUINAL FOLD Fold connecting paramesonephric mesentery to ventral body wall; contains the gubernaculum

INTERMEDIATE MESODERM Subdivision of the somite, between paraxial and lateral plate mesoderm

INTERVILLOUS SPACE Labyrinthine space in which the villi are suspended; is filled with maternal blood

INTRAEMBRYONIC MESODERM *See* Embryonic mesoderm

LABIOGINGIVAL SULCUS Groove between lip and gum

LABIOSCROTAL FOLDS Paired folds that form the scrotum (male) or labia majora (female)

LACUNAE Blood-filled spaces created by erosion of maternal sinusoids by the trophoblast

LANUGO The first, fine coat of body hair

LENS PLACODE Ectodermal precursor of the lens

LENS VESICLE Derived from lens placode, forms the lens

LIMB BUD Earliest rudiment of the limb

LIMB PLATE Expanded extremity of limb bud

LINGUOGINGIVAL SULCUS Groove between tongue and gum

LIQUOR FOLLICULI Fluid in antrum of graafian follicle

MALE PRONUCLEUS The head of the spermatozoon at fertilization

MANDIBULAR ARCH The first branchial arch

MATERNAL (PLACENTAL) COTYLEDONS Islands of placenta created by the placental septa

MAXILLARY PROCESS Process of mandibular arch extending rostral to stomodeum

MEATAL PLATE Ectodermal plate that will break down to create external acoustic meatus

MEROMELIA Partial absence of a limb

MESENCEPHALON The midbrain vesicle

MESENCHYME Undifferentiated mesoderm (embryonic and extraembryonic)

MESODERM *See* Embryonic mesoderm; Extraembryonic mesoderm

MESONEPHRIC DUCT Duct of the mesonephros; in males, forms ductus deferens

MESONEPHROS Temporary kidney formed by the intermediate mesoderm; in males, forms efferent ductules of testis

METANEPHRIC CAP Cells of the intermediate mesoderm that collect around the ureteric bud; forms the nephrons

METANEPHROS The permanent kidney

METENCEPHALON Rostral part of hindbrain; forms pons and cerebellum

MIDGUT (EMBRYONIC) The gut at the level of the vitelline duct; forms the definitive midgut (from point of entry of bile duct to distal part of transverse colon)

MORULA Solid sphere of cells produced by cleavage of the ovum

MYELENCEPHALON Caudal part of hindbrain; forms medulla oblongata

MYOTOME Subdivision of the somite; forms the striated muscles of the trunk

NEURAL ARCH Mesenchymal arch surrounding the neural tube

NEURAL CREST Crest of neural fold; forms the neural crest epithelium

NEURAL FOLDS Ectodermal folds in floor of amniotic sac; precursors of the nervous system

NEURAL PLATE Slipper-shaped ectoderm of the neural folds

NEURAL TUBE Ectodermal tube formed by union of neural folds; forms the nervous system

NEURECTODERM The ectoderm of the neural folds

NEURENTERIC CANAL Passage from yolk sac to amniotic sac through primitive node

NEUROBLAST Parent cell of a neuron

NEUROMERES Segmental zones of high mitotic activity in the neural tube

NEUROPORES Temporary openings at each end of the neural tube

NONDISJUNCTION Failure of separation of a pair of autosomes or sex chromosomes during mitosis or meiosis

NOTOCHORD (DEFINITIVE) Rodlike rostral extension from primitive node, after separation from the endoderm

NOTOCHORDAL PROCESS Rostral extension from primitive node, incorporated into endoderm

OLIGOHYDRAMNIOS Deficiency of amniotic fluid

ONTOGENY The complete developmental history of the individual

OOCYTE Precursor of the ovum

OOGENESIS Development of the ovum

OOGONIA Primordial female germ cells

OPTIC RECESS Ectodermal outgrowth of forebrain; forms optic nerve and retina

ORAL MEMBRANE Area of adhesion of ectoderm to the prochordal plate, rostral to the notochordal process

ORGANOGENESIS Formation of an organ by the assembly of tissues of different kinds

OTIC PLACODE Ectodermal precursor of the otocyst

OTOCYST Precursor of the inner ear

OVULATION Liberation of the secondary oocyte from the ovary

OVUM The mature female gamete

OVUM, PERIOD OF The time from fertilization to completion of implantation, *i.e.,* the first two weeks of development

PARAMESONEPHRIC DUCT Duct formed in the intermediate mesoderm beside the mesonephros; forms epithelium of uterine tubes and uterus

PARAXIAL MESODERM Embryonic mesoderm adjacent to notochord; undergoes segmentation to form somites

PARTHENOGENESIS Cleavage of an unfertilized ovum; can be readily produced in amphibia

PARTURITION Birth

PERIVITELLINE SPACE Space between oocyte (or ovum) and zona pellucida

PHALLUS Precursor of penis or clitoris

PHARYNGEAL ARCHES *See* Branchial arches

PHARYNGEAL GROOVES *See* Branchial grooves

PHARYNGEAL POUCHES *See* Branchial pouches

PHARYNX (EMBRYONIC) The part of the embryonic foregut enclosed by the branchial arches

PLACENTA The organ of fetomaternal gaseous and metabolic exchange

PLACENTA PRAEVIA Placenta attached to the lower uterine segment; may extend to the cervix

PLACENTAL BARRIER (MEMBRANE) Partition between mother and fetus, comprising fetal capillary endothelium and the chorion

PLACENTAL COTYLEDON *See* Maternal cotyledon

PLACENTAL SEPTA Noneroded decidual partitions, coated with trophoblast, dividing the placenta into maternal (placental) cotyledons

POLAR BODIES Minute cells extruded from the oocyte during meiosis

PRIMARY PALATE The median palatal process

PRIMARY VILLUS Villus composed only of trophoblast

PRIMITIVE NODE Expanded rostral end of primitive streak

PRIMITIVE PIT Cavity in primitive node, leading to notochordal canal

PRIMITIVE STREAK Linear zone of cell migration from the ectoderm to form the embryonic mesoderm

PRIMORDIAL GERM CELL Earliest precursor of the gamete

PRIMORDIUM Bud, or early rudiment

PROCESSUS VAGINALIS Peritoneal process extending to the scrotum

PROCHORDAL PLATE Endodermal thickening rostral to the notochordal process

PROCTODEUM Depression external to the cloacal membrane

PROGRESS ZONE Mitotic mesoderm deep to apical ectodermal ridge

PRONEPHROS Earliest kidney rudiment; persists in some fishes

PRONUCLEUS *See* Female pronucleus; Male pronucleus

PROSENCEPHALON Forebrain vesicle

RATHKE'S POUCH Primordium of anterior and middle lobes of hypophysis

RHOMBENCEPHALON Hindbrain vesicle

RHOMBIC LIP Margin of alar lamina of rhombencephalon

ROSTRAL MESODERM The embryonic mesoderm rostral to, and beside, the oral membrane

SCLEROTOME One of the three subdivisions of the somite; enters into formation of the vertebral column

SECONDARY PALATE Portion of palate formed from fused lateral palatal processes

SECONDARY VILLUS Villus composed of trophoblast with core of extraembryonic mesoderm

SEGMENTATION OF THE MESODERM Formation of somites from the paraxial mesoderm

SEGMENTATION OF THE OVUM Cleavage

SEPTUM TRANSVERSUM Transverse mesodermal partition between pericardium and vitelline duct (after formation of head fold)

SINUS VENOSUS Chamber receiving the vitelline, umbilical, and cardinal veins

SOMATIC MESODERM Portion of lateral plate external to embryonic coelom

SOMATOPLEURE Somatic mesoderm together with related ectoderm

SOMITE PERIOD The 20th to 30th days of gestation, during which the somites appear

SOMITES Segmental cell blocks formed from paraxial mesoderm

SPERMATOGENESIS Development of spermatozoa

SPERMIOGENESIS Maturation of spermatozoa from spermatids

SPLANCHNIC MESODERM Portion of lateral plate medial to embryonic coelom

SPLANCHNOPLEURE Splanchnic mesoderm together with related endoderm

STOMODEUM Depression external to the oral membrane

STRATUM GRANULOSUM The many layers of polygonal cells surrounding the maturing oocyte

SUCCENTURIATE LOBE Accessory lobe of placenta

SULCUS LIMITANS Groove between alar and basal plates

SYNCYTIOTROPHOBLAST Syncytial layer of trophoblast

SYNDACTYLY Incomplete separation of fingers

TAIL FOLD The caudal body fold

TELENCEPHALON The cerebral vesicles

TERATOLOGY The study of malformations

TERATOMA Tumor containing derivatives of two or three germ layers

TERMINAL VILLUS Final subdivision of a branch villus

TERTIARY VILLUS Villus containing fetal blood vessels

THECAL GLAND Estrogen-secreting gland surrounding individual ovarian follicles

TOOTH GERM The dental sac together with its contents

TRILAMINAR EMBRYONIC DISK Disk-shaped embryo comprising ectoderm, mesoderm, and endoderm

TROPHOBLAST The cells making up the wall of the blastocyst; give rise to syncytiotrophoblast, cytotrophoblast, extraembryonic mesoderm, and amnion

TRUNCUS ARTERIOSUS Outflow channel of primitive heart

TUBAL GESTATION Implantation and development in the uterine tube

TUBERCULUM IMPAR Temporary swelling in the center of the developing tongue

UMBILICAL CORD The connection between fetus and placenta

UMBILICUS Site of attachment of umbilical cord to body wall

UROGENITAL FOLDS Elevations flanking the urogenital groove; form spongy urethra (male) and labia minora (female)

UROGENITAL GROOVE Midline trough between urogenital folds

UROGENITAL MEMBRANE Ventral subdivision of cloacal membrane

UROGENITAL SEPTUM Coronal partition containing the paramesonephric ducts; in the female, forms the broad ligaments of the uterus

UROGENITAL SINUS Ventral subdivision of the cloaca

URORECTAL SEPTUM Mesodermal septum dividing the cloaca into rectum and urogenital sinus

VAGINAL PLATE Epithelial plate derived from paramesonephric and urogenital sinus epithelium; hollows out to form the vagina

VELAMENTOUS INSERTION OF THE CORD Attachment of umbilical cord to fetal membranes beyond the placental margin

VELLUS Coarser hair which replaces lanugo after birth

VERNIX CASEOSA Cheesy covering of newborn infant, consisting of desquamated periderm and sebaceous secretion

VESICULAR FOLLICLE *See* Graafian follicle

VILLUS *See* Primary villus; Secondary villus; Tertiary villus

VITELLINE MEMBRANE Plasma membrane of the oocyte (later, of the ovum)

WHARTON'S JELLY The mucoid matrix of the umbilical cord

YOLK SAC Vesicle formed by the endoderm

YOLK SAC REMNANT Portion of the yolk sac extruded from the embryo

ZONA PELLUCIDA Hyaline layer between oocyte (later, ovum) and corona radiata

ZYGOTE Unicellular organism formed by union of male and female gametes

index

Individual arteries, bones, muscles, nerves, and veins are listed under these respective headings.